Dr Cherie Martin was born in South Africa, where she qualified as a doctor. She now lives in Glasgow, and practises as a therapist. As the founder of Weigh Ahead, a British organization which offers seminars and workshops in her methods, she has given hope and inspiration to many. She is married, and has one young son.

DR CHERIE MARTIN

NATURALLY SLIM

Without Dieting

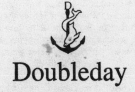

Doubleday

LONDON · NEW YORK · TORONTO · SYDNEY · AUCKLAND

TRANSWORLD PUBLISHERS LTD
61–63 Uxbridge Road, London W5 5SA

TRANSWORLD PUBLISHERS (AUSTRALIA) PTY LTD
15–25 Helles Avenue, Moorebank, NSW 2170

TRANSWORLD PUBLISHERS (NZ) LTD
3 William Pickering Drive, Albany, Auckland

DOUBLEDAY CANADA LTD
105 Bond Street, Toronto, Ontario M5B 1Y3

Published 1996 by Doubleday
a division of Transworld Publishers Ltd
Copyright © 1996 by Dr Cherie Martin

A catalogue record for this book is available
from the British Library.
ISBN 0385 405286

Printed in Great Britain by
Cox & Wyman, Reading, Berkshire.

For Philip and Alan, and in memory of Stephen

Acknowledgements

I would like to thank my cousin, Maureen Kark, who is the author of the Weight Winners programme in South Africa. She is the inspiration behind many of my favourite elements in the programme, including the hunger flow chart, the idea that we become unconsciously skilled and of course the group meal.

I would also like to thank all the American authors in the field whose work I have admired, in particular, Bob Schwartz and Geneen Roth. I discovered Bob Schwartz's book *Diets Don't Work* in 1985 and reading it came as an enormous revelation to me, which helped me escape from my own personal dieting nightmare. I only came across Geneen Roth's books in 1990, but I wish I had discovered them a lot sooner. I would especially like to thank her for telling me about the quiet little voice which tells me to stop eating when I have had enough, and for explaining that 'compulsion is despair on the emotional level'.

I would never have been able to finish the book without the support, encouragement and skilled editing of Marianne

Velmans. She has contributed something to every page of this book, and it was only after she had drawn through, scratched out and filled in other words that my ideas and stories flowed freely and easily. I am indebted to her.

I am grateful to Philip, who encouraged me and told me not to give up, and for laughing and crying with me and for so much more; to my mother for making thousands of cups of tea and washing loads of dishes after each meal, but especially for being with Alan and me in the lonely times; to Jeremy Kingston for his story, his friendship and for providing a place to stay; to Helen Mitchell for our wonderful friendship and our illuminating talks together; to Geoffrey Durham and Shirley Kambule; to Henk Scheepers, June Zats and Gladys Goodman; to my new family, Peter, Joan, Jacki and Timothy; to every single person who works at Corseford School; to my sisters, who live far away but have both been here when I really needed them; to Barbara for the understanding, space and love which absolutely saved my life, and to Christine Haig and Joyce Glasswell for their help in running Weigh Ahead.

Finally, I want to thank every person who has attended my groups and workshops. Your courage, your anger, your love, your tears and laughter; your stories made me think and think, and helped me to develop and focus my theories and ideas. This is *your* book; thank you all.

Author's Note to the Male Reader

I know that men as well as women are subjected to a lot of pressure by society to look thin, and that there are many men who have problems with overeating and dieting. I hope that this book will be of value to them, but I would like to apologize in advance for the fact that I quote from more female case histories than male ones. Most of my groups have been filled by women, probably because society has identified weight as a female problem. But the courageous men who have attended the groups and workshops, although often conspicuously in the minority, have always made an invaluable contribution to our discussions, and I am grateful to them for providing their unique perspective.

Contents

Preface

Everybody says I was such a beautiful baby. Huge blue eyes and a curly mop of brown hair.

I imagine that within a few hours of my birth I experienced a strange sensation in my stomach. As this new feeling intensified I felt scared and uncomfortable, so I cried. My mother breast-fed me and not only did the hunger pangs go, the lovely warm liquidy glow which filled my stomach left me feeling utterly contented. For the first few days of my life the whole process was so satisfying. I got hungry, I ate, I slept, I woke hungry again. Life felt utterly blissful.

Then we returned home from the hospital and everything changed.

I was the result of an unplanned pregnancy eight years after they had given the baby cot and pram away. My parents were struggling to make their failing business survive and my three elder sisters were already all clamouring for the little love and attention that there was available. The family of five had got used to functioning as a unit and there was very little time or energy left for this new and intrusive baby.

My mother fitted in my feeding at a gallop. The only time I ever really had with her was when she was feeding me. In order for me to receive love, then, I had to be eating. That is what I was taught so that is what I learned.

My blue eyes seemed to get bigger and my hair curlier as I grew through my toddler years. Despite the stress in my family I was a warm, vibrant and outgoing child. I would chat happily to strangers and was never scared of new situations.

My father really loved it when I ate a lot. He would speak with pleasure about my big appetite and how I always asked for second helpings. He loved eating, and food was always the most important part of any day or outing.

In contrast my mother and my sisters all were really worried about their weight, so they were constantly trying out the different diets that were around. I soon became aware that it was very important to dress a certain way. The aim was not only to look good but also to look thin. It was cause for great unhappiness if clothes had to be bought in a bigger size and a total calamity if something bought the year before was now too small.

I remember one year during a holiday I had spread a large piece of bread with butter, then apricot jam, and covered that with a design of Cheddar cheese. I went into the playroom where my sisters were, and I was pounced on – 'That's disgusting, each bite of cheese is 30 calories, so that is 30, 60, 90 . . . 210 calories just for the cheese. You are going to get so fat.' Five minutes later I was standing over the rubbish-bin cramming my sandwich into my mouth before they could come in and make me throw it away.

I remember going to the movies and standing with my family at the sweet counter. I felt really excited as my dad said, 'You can each choose an ice-cream and a sweet.' The usual chorus started: 'Dad, that's disgusting . . .' 'All that sugar, Alec, you cannot give these kids sweets, all you ever think about is food.' My father buys himself a huge Mars bar, and I get a small carton of Smarties. The atmosphere of disapproval is palpable. I try and slip the Smarties in without anybody seeing them. I feel bad for wanting them.

Such confusing messages: Eat a lot, really a lot, when Daddy is around – he really likes that. When Mum and sisters are around, eat only when they cannot see, sneak into the kitchen and quickly and quietly finish the leftovers. Offer to make tea so that you can steal some food without being watched by cold, judgemental eyes. That is what I was taught so that is what I learned.

When I was five years old we moved to a new town. I became friendly with Rana, who was my age and our new neighbour. I stayed over for dinner one night and could not believe my eyes. Mounds of roast potatoes, hot and crunchy, with dinner. Ice-cream, as much as we wanted, for dessert. I stood in the middle of their huge warm kitchen with bread in the bread-bin, lots of cake and biscuits in the tin. It was the first time I realized not everybody ate in the same way as my family did. I feel a shudder of unease now, as I remember.

A huge round black table, cold and uncomfortable. Dry grilled chicken and boiled vegetables. Five people much older than me all talking about things I couldn't understand. Telling me to shut up when I asked. Cold and unwelcoming family, low-fat food. An empty place beginning to form inside of me, an empty place that only seemed to fill when I was eating.

It was inevitable, I suppose, that food would take on an extraordinary presence in my life, and that I should begin to overeat and gain too much weight. And then as soon as I was overweight it was inevitable that I should be put on a diet.

I was twelve when I went to Weight Watchers for the first time. I do not remember ever thinking or worrying about my weight before that. I went to school each morning, and I used to spend most afternoons at the swimming-pool, in my favourite blue swimsuit, with my friends. We would run and tumble over each other to get to the ice-cream van when we heard its distinctive music begin to play. There would be a happy silence as we began licking around the bottom of the cone to catch the bits that had already melted in the hot, lazy African sun. I remember how we would all queue, on Tuesday afternoons, for huge helpings of fish and chips at the shop on Robinson Avenue, as we waited for our speech and drama class to begin. We usually spoke and giggled about boys, between mouthfuls. I had a crush on Arnold and made sure he knew about it.

Then it started. I remember the pink folder my Weight Watchers counsellor gave me, which was supposed to record the eleven pounds I was told to lose. I remember measuring and weighing every bit of food that I ate. I remember the embarrassment of queuing up to be weighed with a line of ladies.

I followed the diet exactly as I was told, though, and began to lose weight. I didn't quite notice it then, but my life really changed over those weeks. When my friends ran to the ice-cream van I stayed behind. At dinner-time I ate what I was allowed, then sat and watched my dad have second helpings. He no longer asked me to accompany him on our little 'eating outings', and I missed that. I felt hungry. When we went out I politely refused anything not allowed on my diet, and felt cut off from the other people there, as if I had suddenly got some sort of disease. I missed my secret visits to the kitchen; food had become my only friend at home and now I felt all alone.

The empty feeling inside grew a little bigger.

I reached my goal weight, and my mother and I went shopping for clothes. We bought tight denim jeans, a mini-skirt, and several brightly coloured and skimpy T-shirts. My mother said, 'You see, when you are thin, *everything* looks nice on you.' In fact, many people commented on how good I was looking, and they congratulated me on my weight loss. My group at Weight Watchers applauded when our leader announced that I was now a life member. Everybody seemed so happy that I had lost weight. Everybody that is, except me. 'If everybody tells me I look good now,' I reasoned, 'then I must have looked bad before.' I felt uneasy, embarrassed. I also felt vulnerable, and exposed. My thinness made me feel as if I was naked in my clothes. I had got used to my extra eleven pounds around me and I did not feel as if I fitted into this new body.

I followed the maintenance programme, but a few months later I had regained all the weight I had lost, plus an additional three pounds. My WW counsellor said, 'You are fatter than when you started here, you must go back on the diet.'

I got out my food scale, mixed a pint of water into the correct amount of powdered skimmed milk and started again. But everything was different now. The diet seemed so difficult to follow. I hated trying to make one teaspoon of margarine spread over a whole slice of toast. I hated the feeling of being left out as I ate an apple and watched my friends eat chips in Robinson Avenue. I began to dream about chocolate and pudding. I began to fantasize about a world where food was freely available.

As I think back on all those changes now, I realize that the biggest change was in the way I felt about myself. I weighed only three pounds more than when I began dieting, but I felt totally different. I began making excuses not to go swimming with my friends. How could I? If Arnold saw the mounds of fat sticking out of my blue swimsuit he would hate me. I felt as if I could hide under my school uniform, but if I stripped off, everybody would see that I was a failed Weight Watcher. Everybody would see that I was fat.

I began to spend more afternoons alone. I promised myself that I would go out into the South African sunshine and have fun with my friends again. When I got thin.

Three years later, I had reached my goal twice, given up the diet midway through my third attempt, and now I was due to rejoin Weight Watchers for the fourth time. I no longer had eleven pounds to lose in order to reach my goal, but seventeen, so I was much too embarrassed to return to my original Weight Watchers group. I joined a group in a different area; I thought perhaps it would be the inspiration I needed. It wasn't. I lost weight really slowly, and when I began to regain what I had lost, I decided that I had better try another diet. So I did, and then I tried another and then another. The first diet I tried was to eat half a grapefruit before each meal: the book I read said the enzymes in the grapefruit would burn up everything I ate. Unfortunately the crisps and chocolate from the school tuckshop seemed immune from these magic enzymes, and when the seventeen pounds turned to twenty, my mother took me to buy bigger school uniforms. Then my friend Jenny told me that she lost ten pounds by eating apples and water during the day, and cabbage soup at night. On the sixth day of this regime I ate three apples and drank three glasses of water for breakfast, but within ten minutes of our first lesson, which was English literature, I was squirming. Gaseous eruptions from both ends of me threatened to punctuate each line that our teacher read. I spent the rest of the miserable day close to a toilet, and I ate no apples, or cabbage for that matter, for months afterwards.

I tried so many diets: the Scarsdale, the Beverly Hills, the Cambridge; the grape cure, the seven-day-health diet, the chocolate lover's diet. Each time I lost weight initially, then put back what I had lost plus an extra few pounds. As I played the diet-get-thin-then-get-fat game I became more and more obsessed with it. I no longer cared about romance, or my schoolwork. All I cared about was how much I ate and how much I weighed. During my teenage years, when all my friends were experimenting with boys, clothes and holidays, the first thought that I woke up with each morning was how fat I was. The last thought that I went to sleep with at night was how much or how little I had eaten that day. I lost and regained literally hundreds of pounds. The same pounds, over and over again, in an endless, vicious cycle.

I was really unhappy, and each time I looked for help for my unhappiness, I was told to lose weight – when you are thin, then you will be happy. That sentence, which now makes absolutely no sense to me, was something I firmly believed in, and I lived my life by it. I started each new diet with burning enthusiasm – this was going to be the diet to beat all the others, this time I was really going to lose weight and keep it off for ever. I never did. Every single diet ended with me regaining all the weight I had lost, plus a few pounds extra. What I did lose, I had not intended to lose – I lost time, I lost energy, I lost me.

Every birthday wish, every new year's resolution, was '*I must lose weight.*' I felt so fat, and I really believed that when I was thin I would be happy. When I was thin my whole life would change, I would find the perfect outfit, the perfect boy, the perfect relationship. Every single problem would be solved. When I was thin.

A week after I turned sixteen I came home from school one afternoon and ate a diet salad. Tomato, lettuce and cucumber, with 120 grams of tuna in brine. I took a Diet Coke out of the fridge and then stopped in front of the swing door which led out of the kitchen into the house. The corridor to my bedroom was long and lonely. No one to talk to, nothing to do. I was rooted to that spot on the floor. We had guests over the weekend, and I remembered where I had seen my mother hide the chocolate cake she had baked. I began to sway – lonely corridor or lovely chocolate cake. Lonely, lonely corridor or . . . I dived into the cupboard, feeling slightly shaky. I opened the cake tin and broke off a wedge of dark crumbly icing. It tasted so good. Tomorrow, I thought, tomorrow I will go back on my diet. I got out a dessert plate, cut a huge wedge of cake, poured cream over it and gobbled it down in huge mouthfuls. As I ate I began to calm down. I only stopped eating when I was really full; I felt sleepy, and I hated myself a little more. Tomorrow, I promised myself, tomorrow I would follow the diet.

That binge was the first of many, as a war began to rage inside me. A painful, all-encompassing battle that would last for years. On the one side was the side of me that really wanted to lose weight. A side that believed that to diet was to win, to diet was to clean out cupboards, to finish outstanding chores and to be in control. Then there was the opposing side, a side that needed to eat, that just wanted to eat. All the time.

Food had become the centre of my life. I so desperately wanted to lose weight and yet I needed to anaesthetize myself in food. I wanted to escape and for the few moments that I was eating I could numb myself. Whenever I had a moment spare then I wanted food. I lived and judged my life by the impossible barometer of eating or not eating.

Food had become my lover, friend and mother. I could no longer relate to people, I related to food. I never realized it then, but my childhood had left me with an intense, desperate longing for love. I longed to be thin. I was lonely for love and all I had was chocolate, which was not allowed. I was desperate for a change in the way I was living, so I repeatedly tried to change something about my life. Unfortunately, the very thing I did to try and change would always make me sink deeper into unhappiness. I always tried a new diet.

After high school, I spent a year living with my sister in California. It was meant to be a wonderful opportunity. I was to spend two semesters at UC Berkeley and experience Californian university life, before taking up the place I had been offered at medical school in Johannesburg. The day I arrived, my sister greeted me with the news that she had arranged for me to visit two diet clubs. She said my parents had asked her to help me with my weight problem. Welcome to California, this is the diet we do here. But I had bombed out by then. I could not diet, nor did I even attempt one day of dieting. All I did was eat, from the minute I got up in the morning until the moment each night I collapsed in a food-induced stupor. The only thing I learned really well at Berkeley campus was where all the fastest junk food was available.

This was a crucial time in my development. I was eighteen years old, leaving home and going out into the world for the first time. No longer did I have the regimentation of school and the routine of living in my parents' home. On the surface it seemed as if I had all the skills not only to cope, but also to live a very successful life: straight A scholar, head girl, medical student. Who would have thought there were any problems?

All those things, however, were only on the surface. The empty place inside had become so enormous that it had taken over, and I had become very insecure. I would never initiate a conversation or take risks. I was scared of relationships. I was distanced from my body, and my sexuality.

If you were to meet my mother, my father and my sisters you would probably like them; I hope you would think that they were lovely people to know. But when I was a child they seemed united in their continuous, relentless rejection of me – get out the way Cherie, you are so stupid Cherie, go to your room and leave us alone, no, you can't come with us. No. Stupid. Nuisance. Get away. Go away.

Because my family had been hostile and unwelcoming, I grew up thinking that the world around me was hostile, and full of enemies. And I was frightened. It was only years later that I came to understand that sometimes we do things totally unconsciously, that is, without knowing we are doing them. My fear prompted a strong unconscious need to protect myself. So I did, I built a solid, protective house of fat around myself. In my conscious life I was continuously thinking about food and being thin, but unconsciously I needed to be fat. I equated fat with protection, a barrier against the world.

When I returned from the States I weighed 205 pounds. Diary entry:

Dear Cherie, Happy Shitty 1977. You have just spent a year in America and you have gained five stone, would you like to tell me how you feel about that?

I don't feel as if this fat body is mine. My legs rub together when I walk. My stomach hangs out. I hate this fat, I hate it. I wish I could take a knife and rip it off me, out of me.

*I wake up in the morning and crawl into whatever clothes
will fit me. I try and cover myself with baggy clothes. I wear
the same clothes over and over again. I catch a glimpse of
myself in the mirror and I want to shriek. I want to know
who that revolting fat person is.*

*I avoid people who have not seen me since I gained weight.
Of course they will notice how fat I am. When I do see somebody I haven't seen for a long time then I want to crawl inside myself; I am quiet or I begin making excuses as to why
I have gained weight. I squirm with embarrassment, I wish
I could hide, I wish I could be a woodworm and crawl right
inside the biggest curl of wood and sleep, for ever.*

Being fat makes me ashamed to be alive.

*I exist in the fat and it conceals me, conceals my unhappi-
ness, my fear and my pain. My fat conceals who I really am.
Being fat keeps me living but dead. Being fat ensures that
everything I do is tarnished with the fatness. It is like walking
on broken legs. It is an all-encompassing feeling. I feel fat.*

*Every single part of every day of every feeling is entombed
into one thought, one existence.*

*How am I today? Well, the same as every day. I feel
fat, thank you.*

The first weekend home was my cousin's engagement party, and
I had to face the entire family. I tried to think of an excuse for
not going to the party, but my parents insisted. It was excruciating. We arrived at the party early, so I went into my cousin's
room where she, my aunt, and all her sisters were getting dressed
for the party. My aunt drew in her breath when she saw me, and
they all exchanged amused glances. They hardly waited until I
left the room before they began discussing me, and I heard it all,
every word. 'How can someone be so fat? Did you see how much
weight she has put on? My goodness, talk about waddling!' I
can still hear the sound of the snigger in their voices, and I can
still feel the shame that rushed through my entire body. I ran
outside, tears of humiliation flowing. 'I'll show them,' I fiercely

told myself. 'I will get thin, I will diet and show them that I am a good person. No one will laugh at me again. I will get thin.'

I immediately began the diet which was currently in fashion. A diet doctor had come to town who was producing miracle results. He gave a series of talks to groups of around fifty people at a time. Dr Jack was really charismatic and inspiring and he sold us his method. For a year I ate 500 calories a day and took the appetite suppressants and diuretics he prescribed. I did not go out unless I could take the prescribed food with me. Every time I stood up from sitting I felt dizzy. I felt headachy and tired, my mouth was constantly dry and my tongue felt swollen, as if it did not fit into my mouth, but I never once 'cheated'. I was determined to weigh 128 pounds, and I lost five stone to get there. This time I celebrated my thinness. I covered up how vulnerable I was feeling by wearing my body like a trophy. I went out and bought designer jeans and had a new haircut. I was thin, thin, thin. I walked around being thin. I was still obsessed with my weight. Instead of thinking about how fat I was, I was thinking about how thin I was. It is almost the same thing.

After the initial excitement had died down, I began to see that being slim was not all sunshine and roses. In essence my life had not changed. Inside I still carried a childhood full of unhappiness. All my problems were not suddenly solved. I felt lonely inside when I was overweight and I felt just as lonely when I was slim. Being slim just did not live up to expectations. The strict control I had braced myself with since the engagement party began to fade, and I began to gain weight. I never allowed myself to get as fat as I had done in America, however. Whenever my weight reached 170 pounds, I would go back on the diet.

I continued to follow Dr Jack's diet on and off right through medical school. Two pieces of fruit, one slice of bread, and two meals consisting of 80 grams (raw weight) of protein and a cup of steamed veg or salad. When I was following the diet, I never wavered. I would not eat one lettuce leaf above the prescribed formula. When the diet was over I was always careful with my eating to begin with, but the pounds I had lost would invariably begin to creep back on. Initially I would pretend not to notice that I was choosing only the loose clothes from my wardrobe. Then, inevitably, the day would come when I would look in the mirror and see that I was fat. Again. As I began thinking about starting the diet again, I would begin to really overeat, and binge, all in preparation for the diet to follow.

It was while I was completing my sixth and final year at medical school, thirteen years after my first diet, that I began to see a way out of my diet nightmare. I was browsing in a bookshop, and as I looked across a shelf the title of a book stood out and drew me immediately. It was called *Diets Don't Work*, by Bob Schwartz.

I skipped lectures that afternoon and avidly read every word. I got outraged as I read about the multi-million-dollar diet industry that would like to keep us dieting. I was amazed to read *that only two out of every hundred people are successful at dieting*. I wept as I realized that it wasn't my fault. The years of eating misery had started because when I went on that first diet, I had started down a road which would lead me further and further away from what I really wanted. While I was searching for freedom from my food and weight obsession, constantly being on a diet only caused an increase in my food and weight obsession. A sense of relief poured over me, as I read the book. Suddenly I saw that there was a way out. At last.

The idea explained in the book was that we should model our eating patterns on those of normal people who had no need to diet. People who had never had a weight problem in their lives. Like them we should learn to eat when we were hungry, eat exactly what we felt like eating, and then stop eating when we were satisfied.

Even though I was excited about beginning this new way of eating, I felt terrified to give up dieting. I had a freezer full of pre-measured 80 gram packets of meat and chicken breast, ready for the next time I began Dr Jack's diet. According to Schwartz, if I was to eat as a naturally thin person I was to empty my freezer of diet food, and fill it with ice-cream, apple pies and pizzas, all the foods I loved.

The only life I knew beyond dieting was bingeing, so when I thought of having my cupboards and shelves filled with food I was terrified. Surely I would just eat and eat until everything I had bought was all gone. I was desperate, though, and that desperation made me decide to at least give it a try. I had nothing to lose. I decided to eat when I was hungry and eat exactly what I wanted, for four months, just to see what would happen.

The first task was to learn what natural hunger was. I thought I was hungry all the time, but I had confused emotional hunger with true body hunger. I wanted to eat when I was tired, bored, lonely, angry, anxious or confused. I forgot that the only time I should eat was when I was hungry, in my body.

During the first month, I gained weight. When I was hungry, I wanted all the foods that I had never allowed myself while I was dieting. Especially puddings. The pudding part of any restaurant menu had always had a halo around it; that was what I really wanted. I exhausted every kind of variation of apple crumble, and then went on to sticky toffee pudding. Every time I got hungry and asked myself what I really wanted, the answer was always pudding. Until one day when my friend and I were out for lunch and before the menu arrived I realized that I was hungry for tuna salad. I checked myself: it was reminiscent of a diet lunch. But yes, I really wanted a salad, my body was clearly signalling for something healthy, crunchy and fresh. As I began to incorporate healthy food into my meals in among the puddings, my weight stabilized, and then, to my absolute amazement, it began to go down. Here I was not dieting, eating what I wanted, and I was losing weight!

I know you will want to know exactly how much weight I lost. When I read *Diets Don't Work*, I weighed 170 pounds. In the first months after I stopped dieting, I gained ten pounds. Over the next year I lost forty pounds. I was so excited – the magic wand I had been looking for had arrived. But then my enthusiasm for eating *only* when I was hungry began to fade, and my weight began to creep up again. I thought that it was the same old story. I was crushingly disappointed. But it was at this point that the most interesting and the most difficult part of my journey began.

I realized I still had many important lessons to learn. The first was that even though I needed to learn to eat like a naturally slim person, there was a big difference between slim people and me. Naturally slim people eat when they are hungry, *but they do not eat, or want to eat when they are not hungry*. I did. I wanted to eat when I was tired. I wanted to eat when I was lonely. When I was happy, bored, excited. When I had a headache or needed to fill any empty spaces in my day. It was often a big struggle for me to give up eating when I was not hungry. Reaching for food for comfort was a familiar, ingrained habit and I could not lose it in an instant. While I was learning how to not eat when I was not hungry, my weight did fluctuate, up as well as down. However, the long-term trend was always downwards.

Right through this book I have used case histories. On re-reading them I realize that because I have condensed them into this book they often fail to reveal the time and struggle that was involved for each person. And so too with my story. I gave up dieting nine years ago; during that time my son Alan was born prematurely, weighing two pounds. The after-effects of his traumatic first year have left him with cerebral palsy, and he will always be in a wheelchair. When he was two, his father, my darling first husband, Stephen, died very suddenly. I have coped with what happened to me, and I have also expressed my grief with wild fluctuations in my weight. I needed to. There were times when food seemed to be the only thing in the world which could provide comfort, and other times, in my grief, when not eating, and losing weight, brought a semblance of control into my world, which had become chaotic and uncontrollable. My biggest task was to learn not to suppress my feelings in food. To be strong enough to cry when I am sad, to express my anger, and to eat only when I am hungry.

With relief I realize that if I had allowed my obsession with food to continue, I would have lost the essence of who I really am. I am a woman, I am a lovely person to know. I am not my weight or how I look. I have sad times, I have happy times, and I often make mistakes. These times are never governed by how much I weigh or how pretty I look. These times are governed by how I feel. How I feel inside.

I never weigh myself now; my weight probably fluctuates by half a stone, but that does not matter. If you could see me now you would notice that I am smiling as I write; it doesn't matter, I don't mind what I weigh. I am surprised how personal this book has turned out to be, but I realize that by telling you exactly how I resolved my weight problem I can show you how you can overcome yours. It was a journey for me to heal myself, a journey with several turning points.

When I was young, I would dream of the good fairy who would grant me three wishes. My first fervent wish was always that I could eat as much as I wanted and never get fat. Recently I celebrated my thirty-fifth birthday, and I realized that that childish wish had come true: I can eat whatever I want, whenever I am hungry, and I do not mind what my weight is. You can do the same: read this book and see.

PART 1

1

Health Warning – Dieting is Dangerous for Your Health, and It Makes You Fat

'I went on a diet. For a fortnight I forsook food and drink, and at the end of it I had lost fourteen days.'

JERRY LEWIS

'The punishment for eating is the punishment of fat, and dieting's the punishment for that.'

IRENE O'GARDEN

Dear Dr Martin

I heard that you run programmes to help us poor long-suffering dieters. I am aged 48, and at this moment I am carrying 12 stone 7 lb on my 5 foot and seven inches frame. I have been battling for over 30 years with one diet or another. My husband has told me that he is thoroughly bored with the various diets and talk of diets and strange food I make while I am dieting. Quite frankly

I am also sick and tired of dieting, I find the whole business so tedious. I always seem to end up bingeing and in despair. In the newspaper article I read about you it was mentioned that you have lost forty pounds without dieting. Could you tell me how you managed to do that? Could you tell me how you manage to spend your days without overeating? Please send me any information that you have, I enclose a blank cheque to help cover your expenses.

Your sincerely
Carol Stevens (Mrs)

I meet so many different people, all desperate for the same thing: help with their weight problem. Intelligent, successful people who easily manage their jobs, homes and families. People who know all about calories, hidden fats, how to exercise, and how to diet. Famous people, housewives, doctors, managing directors, and students. All different people with the same problem. They feel overfed, overweight and out of control around food.

All these different people have one thing in common. At some point in their lives they went on that first diet. That is what happened every single time.

The minute we go on a diet we begin an unavoidable chain of events. The way we think about food is totally changed, the way our body burns what we eat is slowed down, our self-esteem becomes totally wrapped up in our weight, and, worst of all, we get so caught up in a cycle of dieting or bingeing that we forget how to eat naturally and normally.

I know that diets do work in the short term. If you restrict the amount of calories you take in, you will lose weight, and you will enjoy the initial high of that weight loss. You will feel light and happy as you throw away your hide-away-tent clothes, and shop for new ones.

Inevitably, once the diet is over, things begin to change. In the beginning you only overeat occasionally – a bite or two of chocolate or an extra slice of toast. Then you feel reckless, or anxious, and you have your first whole weekend blowout. While you are overeating, you feel guilty, out of control, but you tell yourself you deserve it, this once. After all, you can always start the diet again.

Tomorrow.

You begin to gain weight, a pound or two at first, then five, and before you know it you have a stone to lose. You keep on planning to start the diet again, you even buy the special low-fat, sugar-free ingredients, but it feels really difficult. One more day, you promise yourself, and then you will definitely start. You get fatter. And so the days turn to weeks, the five pounds turn to six, and then to twelve, and suddenly, you are fat again. With undisguised sarcasm people begin to tell you how well you are looking. You feel ashamed, embarrassed, you begin to crawl about again in your big clothes.

You try and motivate yourself – for that wedding, in twenty-one days' time. Twenty-one days to starve yourself so that you can fit your size 16 body into the size 12 suit you have hanging in your wardrobe. The morning of the first of those twenty-one days, you decide that since twenty days is an even number, you can overeat for just one more day and definitely start again.

Tomorrow.

The time of being thin seems like a dream. You try to remember what happened. The diet was such hard work, so many times you went hungry, and said no to dessert. The trophy size 10 trousers still hang in your wardrobe. What happened? You were thin for a moment, and now you are fat again, fatter than before. What happened?

I'll tell you what happened. Dieting just does not work. Study after study has shown that 98 per cent of people who go on a diet regain the weight they have lost. I find that percentage so amazing that I want to say it again: ONLY TWO OUT OF EVERY HUNDRED PEOPLE WHO DIET ARE SUCCESSFUL IN THE LONG TERM. I have a special gun. Its barrels are 98 per cent loaded. So if we play Russian Roulette you have a 2 per cent chance of surviving when I hold the gun to your head and pull the trigger. Some odds. The same odds apply for successful permanent weight loss by dieting.

Rosemary Conley has sold more than two million books since she launched her fat-free for hips and thighs philosophy, Weight Watchers has hundreds of thousands of members around the world, slimming magazines sell hundreds of thousands of copies, low-fat foods and low-calorie meals are big business. Magazines and newspapers that feature the latest diet on their front cover are guaranteed to sell more copies. The dieting industry is booming!

'Buy-us-and-get-thinner' products surround us: diet pills, exercise videos, powdered meal replacements, slimming aids, fad diets, more, more and more. Figures released by the Economist Intelligence Unit show that as a nation we spent £70 *million* on slimming products in 1993 – almost 20 per cent up on the figure for 1992, and a 100 per cent increase since 1989. In Britain, as many as one woman in four is usually on a diet of some kind, and 90 per cent of all women will have dieted at some point in their lives. We have become desperate and relentless in our pursuit of slimness. We want to be slim, and we keep dieting in order to get slim.

Surely if we are spending all this money we should expect everybody to be getting thinner and thinner? Tom Sanders and Peter Bazalgette, in their book *You Don't Have to Diet*, show that unfortunately the opposite is true. They quote a recent government survey which shows that in 1980 8 per cent of women and 6 per cent of men were obese, and that by 1991 that figure had *doubled* to 16 per cent of women and 13 per cent of men. I really cannot get over this: we have doubled the amount of money which we spend on diet products, and yet we are twice as fat. Obviously we spent money on the wrong products – if diets worked we would all be much thinner, not fatter.

It took years before there was a government health warning on cigarette packets, and it is only very recently that the

information about the danger of dieting
through. A motion was recently tabled in P
curbs on the diet industry, and the advertisi
has been tightened up in relation to ads for s
and diets, especially for young people. Meanw
pouring more money into a multi-billion-poun   ry,
which is of course exactly what the manufactu   want us
to do.

What a good situation for the people who are selling diet
products. I imagine them rubbing their hands with glee, and
congratulating themselves on all the money they have made.
What could be better for them? The fatter everybody gets, the
more new diet products they will sell. Whatever new and fancy
paper the new 'Get Thin' promise is wrapped up in, when we
tear it off we always find the same thing. A diet. And diets just
don't work.

In the next few pages I will describe in detail the damage
that diets can do. My intention is not only to convince you
even further that dieting does not work, but also to help you
understand the chaos that has been caused in your mind and
body by all the years of dieting. Even if you gave up dieting
years ago, it will be useful to understand what happened to you
during the years when you did diet. Only when we understand
exactly what damage has been done can we go ahead and create
new solutions.

1. Diets make you overeat, and binge

It is Friday afternoon and Laura has just arrived home from
work. She has been dieting rigidly for twelve days, a low-cal
shake for breakfast and another for lunch and then 300 calories
for dinner. She has strictly kept to this programme and she feels
really pleased with herself. She also feels hungry, very hungry. A
hunger which extends from her stomach all the way up through

...ck and into her throat. She begins to think about dinner ...d realizes that if she eats her dinner now she will have finished her entire food quota for the day. She decides to quiet down her hunger pangs with a Diet Coke, and a carrot, so that she can save her meal for later.

Then the phone rings. It is her friend, who suggests that they go out for dinner. Laura hesitates – she knows that saying yes to dinner means she cannot stick to her diet. Oh hang, she decides, I will go and then I will start dieting again tomorrow.

Laura starts to run a bath and get her clothes ready, and as she does so she makes several trips into the kitchen, for a biscuit, then bread, then ice-cream. She feels guilty about eating, 'But after all I am really hungry,' she reasons, 'and I won't be able to stick to my diet later, and I will definitely diet tomorrow, definitely.'

On the way home from the dinner Laura thinks about how much she has eaten, and she feels awful. She is so full she could burst. She had begun to feel full after two mouthfuls of her main course, but she carried on eating, through the main course, through the salad. In order to eat the lemon meringue pie she had to take huge deep breaths between bites. She just could not stop. She was angry with herself, but she just kept on promising herself, 'Tomorrow, tomorrow I will diet.'

There is a part of Laura that sees what is happening, that sees what she is doing. If only she would listen she would hear this part of herself speaking in a low and urgent voice: 'Laura, please stop, this has been going on for years and years. The same thing over and over again. The only way you ever give yourself permission to eat is to tell yourself that you will diet on Monday, and because you know that from Monday you will have to survive on low-cal shakes. You never just eat, you always overeat. I wish you could see what you are doing, Laura, you are either sticking to a diet and undereating or you are preparing for the diet tomorrow by overeating. When you are on a diet you feel deprived and depressed and when you break it you feel bloated and hate yourself. You are living a nightmare, Laura, and you keep doing the same thing, over and over. Please stop.'

Unfortunately Laura does not seem to hear this wise inner voice. All she hears is a cruel voice which says, 'Laura, you are revoltingly fat, look at those rolls on your stomach, look how you wobble. You have gone and blown it again – did you see how much you ate tonight? I do not believe that one person could eat all that. You are fat and a failure, and you'd better just do something about your weight. You'd better diet and do it properly this time.'

Laura is not alone. She is one of the many thousands of us who are in a self-defeating cycle. We diet because we feel overweight, and it is that very dieting that drives us to overeat between diets, and makes us fatter.

It is only quite recently that various researchers have started to ask the question: Does dieting cause overeating? One of the experiments they used to investigate this was to give one group of volunteers a high-calorie snack followed by a meal, and another group of volunteers a low-calorie snack followed by a meal. The researchers then measured how much each person ate at the meal. Logically we would expect to find that if a person had eaten a high-calorie snack before a meal they would eat less during the meal, and indeed this was found to be true, but *only for people who had never dieted*. For the people in the experiment who were dieters, logic had nothing to do with it. The high-calorie snack actually served as encouragement for them to eat a huge meal. Feeling hungry or full had nothing to do with it. Eating a load of calories meant for them that the diet was blown anyway, so they might as well overeat.

We really need to acknowledge this trap we are in. We think we need to diet because we are overweight. We become overweight because we overeat, and *we overeat because we diet*.

I had been thinking about this strange habit of ours – how we are able to diet for months and months, and then, when we have lost the weight, we are unable to eat without overeating. It seems very strange. People who do not have weight problems only overeat on special occasions, but dieters regularly overeat.

Then one day my son and I were playing with his wind-up toy clown. You insert a key into the clown's back and you turn the key around, and around, tighter and tighter, until eventually you hear a click and the key is ejected. As soon as the key is out, the spring is released, and the clown dances, madly, frenetically. Ho-ho-ho. Then, as his energy supply dwindles, he slows down and his smile droops. He still dances, but he actually begins to look sick, and then he goes slower still, and looks sicker, until he has nothing left, and he stops, dead.

They seemed to me to symbolize why we binge after we diet, that key and that clown. The diet is the winding of the key, and the binge is the dance. The more rigid the diet, the tighter we wind the spring, and the longer the clown will dance his sick dance.

Every time we go hungry while we are surrounded by a sea of food, every time we say no to foods we really want, it is as if we are giving that key one more turn. The more we turn the more the energy builds up inside, until one day the pressure gets too much, and the key will just pop out. Then we will eat frantically. We eat for all the times we have said no in the past, and for all the times we will say no in the future. The binge dance is desperate, we must get everything in quickly before we start winding that key again.

Most diets are followed by a corresponding binge. The binge continues in proportion to how long we dieted, and only stops when we have run out of energy and we have eaten all the food we didn't allow ourselves while we were dieting. Unlike the toy clown, however, we don't laugh. We suffer, and when we stop, we are fat. Again.

Dieting causes bingeing.

The only way to stop bingeing is to stop dieting.

2. Diets Make you Gain Weight

Have you ever noticed that over the years it has become progressively more difficult for you to lose weight? You begin the same diet that you followed successfully last year, but this time your weight loss is much slower and, to add insult to injury, when you stop the diet you gain weight again really quickly. I remember that the first time I went to Weight Watchers I lost weight easily and fast, but after five years of dieting, if I ate the amount of food that was on my original Weight Watchers food plan, I just managed to maintain my weight, not lose weight. Increasingly, the only way I could lose weight was to go on starvation or crash diets. Many of my course participants have bemoaned the fact that they eat much less than their naturally slim friends do, yet they never lose weight, and when they do eat normally, they gain weight really quickly.

This pattern, which occurs in most dieters, can be explained when we look at the method of survival which was evolved by prehistoric man. There were no refrigerators or food preservatives, so he evolved a method to store food which was simple yet effective. He used his body. When food was plentiful, he feasted and built up an extra layer of fat. He then used that extra layer of fat for energy during the long, cold winter months, or at other times when food was in short supply.

Food shortages and famine are due to drought and bad weather conditions; they happened in the past, and they still occur in the Third World countries, or where war breaks out. But in our own wealthy peacetime consumer society, we create our own food shortages. We go on a diet.

Our body does not understand our wish to be a size 10, so when we diet, the only thing that our body registers is that there is a decreasing amount of food coming in. This decrease in food activates our ancient survival mechanisms – it is as if your body rings an alarm bell which says: 'Warning, warning, there is not enough food around. Don't know how long this will last. Quickly start protection mechanisms: slow down, conserve energy, store as much of the food that comes in as fat for the future, and when the fat is stored, hang on to it. Make sure that it lasts as long as possible so that if we starve again we will survive.'

The body achieves this reaction by slowing down our metabolic rate. Metabolic rate is the speed at which we burn food in order to provide energy for us to carry out our daily activities. If the body wants to conserve energy it slows this rate down. We burn the food we eat more slowly, we convert more of the food we eat into fat, and we are slowed down. We move more slowly, we have less energy, we feel tired.

The longer the diet continues, the more efficient the body becomes at storing food. This effect lasts even when we stop dieting, because the body continues to burn food at this slower rate. If a normal-weight person eats a piece of toast they burn it up for energy. If somebody who is a chronic dieter eats toast they immediately store some of the toast as fat for the future.

It really becomes a vicious cycle. Eventually the same amount of food that we used to eat to lose weight becomes the maximum intake of food we can eat to maintain our weight, without gaining. In fact the best way to *gain* weight is to keep on dieting. Dieting followed by bingeing ensures that we keep this cycle going.

Before I thoroughly depress you, I will tell you that there are some immediate steps you can take to start to undo this damage that dieting has done to your metabolic rate. First, never, ever allow yourself to get ravenously hungry. We need to reassure our bodies that there is enough food and that it need not keep stockpiling for the future. If a steady supply of enough food is available, our bodies have no need to store food for future deprivation. If there is a shortage of food, followed by a surplus, our bodies will make sure that they store the surplus for the deprivation to follow.

Second, regular exercise can help restore your metabolic rate to normal – I will discuss this in more detail in Chapter

8, Learning to Love Your Body.

3. Dieting Makes You Obsessed with Food

Last Monday it was an icy cold day. As I was eating and enjoying a bowl of steamy vegetable soup, I became aware of the conversation at the table next to mine. Two women, each nursing a can of Diet Pepsi, spent an entire hour talking about their diet and their weight. 'It's nice to have the list of free foods,' one said, 'so if I am hungry I can have six tomatoes.' 'Apparently we just have to get through the first few weeks, and then it gets a lot easier,' the other replied. Right through the conversation, whenever any plates of food were carried past these two they looked at them longingly. They both looked hungry. I wished they would eat something. I wished for their sakes they would talk about something else. They would both have got a whole lot more out of their conversation.

Dieting changes us. When we are on a diet, we begin to live very differently. Perhaps without even noticing we begin to talk and think a lot about food. We have long conversations about what we are allowed for breakfast, what we are not allowed for lunch. We discuss how to make our allocation of allowed food last longer, and about how we are going to feast when the diet is over. Then we begin to notice people eating in the streets, how wonderful a bakery store smells. We spend increasing amounts of time thinking about our weight and planning what food we are going to eat each day. Eventually we end up preoccupied, obsessed with the very thing we are trying to give up – food.

Now you may think it is a good idea to be obsessed with food, because then you can remember to watch carefully what you eat. Unfortunately it has the opposite effect. When thoughts about food are always creeping through our minds, we constantly reach for food when we are not hungry. Being obsessed with food means that in the middle of our brain there is a box, and inside the box is written 'EAT SOMETHING, HAVE SOME

FOOD'. This box is filled to overflowing with these words, so any stimulus whatsoever causes the words to spill out into our brains. For example, we may feel sad about something but before the sadness is allowed to come to the surface, the box opens and our obsession interferes and we immediately want to eat. We feel stressed, and food becomes the solution we think of to calm ourselves down. We get lonely, and instead of reaching out to another person, food becomes our unsatisfactory friend. Any feeling, whether it be happy or sad, first passes through the box sitting in our brain, and often gets short-circuited by it. We diet, we become obsessed with food, and then we are stuck, short-circuited. Wherever we go, whatever we do, we hear the message: Eat something, have some food.

A friend of mine went on a diet recently. She had no interest in losing weight, as she has been naturally slim all her life, but she was plagued by recurrent candida (thrush) infections and had read that she could 'starve the candida out of her system' by eliminating all sugar and yeast products from her diet. She phoned me after ten days on her new regime. 'Cherie, it's amazing, I walked past the bakery today, and I actually slowed down. Everything looked so inviting, I took deep breaths just so that I could smell the things inside. The funny thing is that I pass this shop on my way to work every day and previously I hardly even noticed it was there. Now all I can think about are the twisted doughnuts that I saw in the window. I can't stand this! Usually I never want sweet things; now that I am not allowed them, they are all I think about all day.' A few days later Maggie couldn't resist any longer: she went into the bakery and came out with two twisted doughnuts and a loaf of fresh white bread. She ate the doughnuts in huge gulps on the way to her office, and when she got there she pulled off slice after slice of bread and ate until she was satiated. 'I will never do that to myself again,' she told me afterwards. 'I felt like I was turning into a bakery shop junkie.'

Deprivation causes an obsession with forbidden foods and leads to bingeing. All this happened to Maggie after a couple of weeks – just think what would have happened to her after years of dieting!

4. How Are You Today? Fat, Thank You

Diets not only cause us to become obsessed with food, they also encourage us to have an unhealthy focus on how much we weigh. Diet clubs encourage this emphasis. We are applauded when we lose weight and there is no applause if we gain. We are given a goal weight and then we become so fixated on what the scales say that how much we weigh becomes a barometer of how we are feeling. If our weight is down we allow ourselves to be happy, but if the scales measure a weight gain, our world comes crashing down around us.

I love going to the steam baths at my gym. I wrap myself in a big fluffy towel and put my feet up while I read or listen to music. I have never been to the gym without hearing at least one woman comment on her weight. Someone is always noticing or talking about how much weight they have lost or gained.

Then, of course, there are the scales. I see the faces as they step on and step off; I can tell what verdict has been delivered by the Lord Judge, Her Highness the Weighing Machine. If the person has lost weight there is a lightness in their step, but more usually they step off the scales and drag their heavy body away. How many mornings have you woken up feeling happy until . . . you step on the scales. If the needle goes up your day is ruined, ruined.

One day at gym I noticed two friends having an animated, happy conversation. One of them disappeared for a few moments and returned looking absolutely heartbroken: 'I have gained *two* pounds,' she said to her friend. 'Can you believe it, two whole pounds.' Her friend made a few consolatory remarks but soon lost interest. The now-two-pounds-heavier one would not speak about anything else. She analysed her eating over the last few days, and talked about what she was going to do to lose the weight. She did not even notice that her friend had withdrawn and that their previously intimate conversation had become a boring monologue about the two pounds.

If I weigh myself and then drink a litre of water I will gain close to two pounds. When I am premenstrual I can gain much more than that. Yet here was a young woman devastated by what was probably no more than a natural fluctuation in weight. Scales are definitely not an accurate measure of how fat or thin we are, yet we let what the needle on the scale says ruin or make our day. This obsession with how much we weigh can become really severe. I have clients who hop on and off the scale several times a day – before and after each meal, after going to the toilet, with clothes and without clothes. Each time they weigh themselves their mood changes accordingly, in fact their whole day is linked and often ruined by this unhealthy scale-hopping habit.

I spoke to Ray, a neighbour, the other day and asked her how she was. 'Well, I lost two pounds last week but this week my weight has stayed the same,' she answered. 'I didn't ask how your weight was, I asked how you are,' I replied. 'I am really not interested in what you look like – I am interested in what you have been thinking about, in what has been happening in your life. I am interested in you.' For Ray her weight obsession is so much to the fore that she has confused how she is feeling with how much weight she has, or has not, lost.

This weight obsession is fuelled by society's blind verdict that if we have lost weight we are in control, but if we have gained weight we are to be sniggered at and pitied. A large number of people seem to confuse feeling good with feeling thin, and feeling fat with feeling bad. I remember that two years after my first husband, Stephen, died, my grief and depression were at their worst. I could not eat or sleep, and my weight dropped to the lowest it has ever been. My hair was falling out, my skin would bruise if you touched me – and most of the people I encountered told me how *wonderful*

I looked, and what a beautiful figure I had. I was dying and lonely inside, and yet because I was thin the implied comment was that I was doing wonderfully. How we feel inside is how we feel inside. Our external appearance, especially extreme weight fluctuations, may be an indicator of what is going on in our lives, but being thin definitely does not mean that things are going well!

If we gain weight when we are feeling unhappy, it usually means that we need to look at what is happening in our lives – our jobs, our relationships, where and how we are living. Most of us, especially if we have been overweight for a long time, also need to work on improving our self-esteem. If we start paying less attention to how much we weigh and more attention to the way we are living our lives, we will be happier, and we will eat less.

Unfortunately our weight-obsessed society encourages us to focus on losing weight as a cure for all ills. This obsession with our weight is made apparent by how many women, and an increasing number of men, talk about their weight to each other. They explain why their weight is at the level it is, and they discuss other people's weight as if it were a news item. Somehow we have all come to accept that thin is good and fat is bad.

I have often been amazed at the cruel way people comment on each other's weight. We would probably think twice before telling anybody that there was a smear of food on their face, or that there was something green in their nose; yet we all find it totally acceptable to comment on each other's weight. I and many of my clients have been devastated by the comments made by unthinking people. 'My, haven't you grown?' 'Why don't you join Scottish slimmers?' 'I guess you won't want any cakes.' 'My aunt is as big as you.'

5. Naughty but Nice – The Seduction of Forbidden Foods

As we arrived at Craig's fifth birthday party he proudly showed us the fancy remote control car he had received as a gift from his parents. Craig wanted to play with his new car, but his mother said that because only one person could play with it at a time he should wait until later. From that moment on he protested and whined and all he would talk about was the car. His mother tried everything – started the party games, brought in the cake, showed him all the other presents. Craig would not waver, he wanted his new car, and he wanted it now. The more he was told he couldn't have it the more he wanted it. Eventually his mother relented and brought the car downstairs. Craig was delighted, and all his friends gathered around to see him play with his new present – for exactly five minutes. Then all the children, Craig included, lost interest and were off to play another game.

One strange thing about human nature is that we always want what we have been told we cannot have. Things have a strange attraction when we know that they are not allowed. When we look at the diet sheet and see that it says no chocolates, sweets, fats, alcohol, or cakes, those foods immediately become really special. The damage gets worse and worse as we try to satisfy our hunger with a plateful of lettuce while we watch other people feasting on hot puddings and roast potatoes.

The longer we deny ourselves these foods, the more we want them. When we crumple up our diet sheets, previously forbidden foods will be all we want at first. But when we have the freedom to have exactly what we want, their allure will dwindle. When I approach a box of chocolates with the thought, 'I am not allowed this, I shouldn't eat this,' then I am going to want the whole box. The only thing making the chocolate so seductive and powerful is that it is forbidden. And if it is forbidden I may think that I want it, even when I do not really want it. If it is not forbidden then I have the freedom of choice: I can choose to have some chocolate or not have some. My choice, just mine.

6. Dieter's Logic: The Eating Excuses

Perhaps there was a time when you were younger when food was absolutely no issue. It was there to be eaten when you were hungry. A time when you could leave the dinner table without giving a thought to how much or how little you had eaten. A time when you would just stop eating when you had eaten enough. You never spent even one minute thinking about your weight. You sometimes ate just for fun, you sometimes ate a little and sometimes a lot – either way, it was no big deal.

Then the years of dieting and deprivation began. Food was no longer just part of our lives. Rather we placed a whole lot of rules and regulations around our eating. Then because we wanted what we had told ourselves we could not have, we began to bargain with ourselves around food – in fact we collected a whole lot of what I call eating excuses.

I used to be so good at these eating excuses. Long after I gave up dieting I would always eat when I was hungry, but then I often managed to find perfectly good excuses to eat when I was not hungry. Here are some of my own eating excuses, and some shared by participants in my workshops.

Eating now in case I get hungry later
I will be out the whole afternoon and I won't be able to eat anything, so I'll eat something now in case I get hungry later.

Reward for hard work
I have had such a hard day – I worked overtime, did the shopping, came home and did housework. I deserve a treat, a

reward for all that, so I will eat something even though I am not hungry.

Food is love
I need a hug, I need comfort, I need someone to wrap me in a fluffy blanket and make the world go away; so I will make myself a hot drink and a huge sandwich. Anyway food cannot talk back to me, hurt me or leave me.

A shot of energy
I am so tired and I still have so much work to do; I need a cup of coffee and something sweet to perk me up.

Keep eating my pain away
I hurt, I feel really low, so I will try to soothe away the tears and swallow the lump in my throat with piles of food.

Food will calm me down
Stress, stress, so much going on, so much to do and I feel like I am drowning, I really need a lifeboat, and I choose cheese on toast to save me from sinking.

I've started so I may as well finish
I shouldn't really be eating this packet of biscuits but they were quite expensive and it would be a waste to throw them away. I don't want to have to deal with the temptation tomorrow, so I'll quickly eat the whole packet now.

Feast if it is free
Out to a five-course dinner and since somebody else is paying I must eat every last morsel. I don't care that I will leave feeling ill, I must eat everything – and anyway I will start dieting tomorrow.

Tasting my way around the world
My first trip to California, Fiji or Timbuktu – food is part of the fun and I must taste everything I have never eaten before, and since I will never eat it again I must be sure to have lots of it.

I've exercised so I can eat

I did an aerobics class today and I will do one tomorrow, so I will burn off everything I am going to eat tonight.

Swallow my anger

I am *angry*, so angry I could hit something. I don't know what to do with the anger so I will bury it in a mound of carrots and cheese.

Calorie-counting

If I work it out I have only had a thousand calories today so I will eat the cream bun, never mind whether I am hungry or not; I should have thirteen hundred calories a day, so I will eat something now.

Food nostalgia

Oh, I haven't had this kind of pudding since I was a child! I'm not hungry but I remember I used to feel so good when I ate this.

Sleeping pills are bad for you so food will have to do

I can't sleep so I will have a hot milky drink and a biscuit.

I knock myself out of life

Food, the great escape. First the time spent eating, and then the time spent shouting at myself for eating. I don't need to worry about what is going on in my life, I just escape into the oblivion of a weight problem all the time.

Nothing to do, nowhere to go

I am so bored. What will I do? Well, I will just eat something or go out to eat, at least it is something to do.

Food becomes the friend I need

I am lonely, and as my addiction to food has grown so I have withdrawn from other people. At least I have this tub of ice-cream to keep me company.

Self-inflicted punishment

I hate myself, I am guilty and ashamed of who I am, so I

will eat something; who cares if I get fatter, I deserve to be punished so this is how I will punish myself.

Feed a fever and a cold

I don't feel well, I need a good hearty curry to sweat out a cold. I need lots of roughage — six packets of dried fruit!!! I have just recovered from bronchitis and I need to eat lots and lots to keep my strength up. When I am hot I eat cold food and when I am cold I eat hot food. I use food as a medicine for all my body complaints.

The diet starts . . . tomorrow

Tomorrow I will go on the straight and narrow. I can eat now, because tomorrow I will diet.

Even when I stopped dieting I continued to use that last eating excuse, I told myself that it was fine to overeat today because tomorrow I would eat when I was hungry and stop when I was satisfied. This is the old dieters's logic, and it makes no sense. Telling yourself you will deprive yourself tomorrow provides an eating excuse for today.

I know it's stupid, you know it's stupid. Looking back over these excuses I want to laugh, but they also make me want to cry. They sum up the elaborate deceptions, the lies we dieters have told ourselves over the years. Who is the victim of this deception? Nobody but us.

7. Doing Something About Your Weight Instead of Doing Something About Your Life

Gloria came to see me, desperately unhappy. She blamed the unhappiness on how fat she was. For the first half-hour of her session all she could talk about was how she really had to do something about her weight. I eventually managed to draw her attention away from her weight, and only then did she manage to speak about what was really bothering her.

A colleague at work had mentioned that there was a rumour of six job losses in their company, and she was worried about keeping her job, as she had fallen several weeks behind in doing her reports. She felt that her relationship with her husband was deteriorating. The house was a mess and her car kept stalling in traffic. All this was going on, yet all she could think about was what to do about her weight!

As a result of our conversations over the ensuing weeks, Gloria confronted her husband and they began to work on their relationship. She spoke to her immediate boss at work and was reassured about her job. They also worked on how she could be more efficient at getting her reports done. She hired a cleaner and got her car repaired. While all this was going on she lost a stone in weight without even thinking about it.

In order to feel better we need to work on what is really happening in our lives – if we continue to pour all our energy into dieting and how much we weigh, the vicious cycle continues, and we still haven't changed the real cause of unhappiness in our lives. All we have done is fail at another diet.

8. When I Am Slim, My Life Will Be Perfect

When I am slim I will:

> Go swimming.
> Buy new clothes.
> Change my job.
> Find the perfect partner.
> Leave my husband.
> Start living.

Sounds familiar? So many people I meet are fixed in the belief that when they become slim all their problems will be solved, and they will be happy.

Being slim can make you feel lighter, more self-confident,

and more comfortable when you are buying clothes, but it cannot solve all your problems. It cannot take away the pain of an unhappy marriage, or the boredom of a dead-end job. Being slim is just being slim, that is all.

When Penny was thirteen her parents got divorced, and soon after her father remarried he severed all connections with Penny, her brother and their mother. Six years later, when Penny was nineteen, she met and married Tom, a man thirteen years her senior. For a brief period the feelings of abandonment that she had felt when her father left were gone.

But it was not long before Penny realized that she had married a cold and critical man. He treated her as if she was his live-in servant. Penny secretly went on the pill, and decided that as soon as she had a job that paid enough for her to support herself, she would leave him. In the meantime she found a way to take the sting out of the cruel way he treated her – she would go into the kitchen and eat something. A chocolate biscuit for sweetness when he shot acid comments at her. A soft cheesy roll to swallow down the lump in her throat. Bowls and bowls of hot creamy rice pudding to keep her company on lonely nights. In fact she began to find all her comfort and solace in food.

When she began to gain weight, Tom ridiculed her. He mocked her about her huge thighs and legs, and scolded her when she became short of breath and could not keep up with him in the street. One night, when they returned from a party, he told her that he was sleeping with other women, but it was her fault because she had let herself get so fat and revolting. Penny hated him. She was even more desperate to leave.

What Tom said about her weight shocked her, though, so she joined a slimming club. It was the first diet she had ever been on, so it worked rapidly and in a few months she had lost most of the weight she had gained during her marriage. Nothing changed. Tom was just as mean to her as he had ever been – she was just as lonely, just as unhappy. She enjoyed wearing slim clothes, and she enjoyed the compliments people gave her about her weight loss – but that wasn't enough to sustain her on her low fat regime. She missed the comfort that food had given her on her alone nights, and she soon began to overeat again.

Penny withdrew more and more into herself; she ate a lot and dreamed a lot. She had confused herself, though, because her dreams were all about becoming slim. In her mind being fat trapped her – she believed she could not do the things she really wanted to do because she was fat. Penny actually believed that fat people did not have the right to do the things that slim people do. She fantasized about how she would live in a lovely flat, change her job, and go swimming three times a week. (She had stopped when her size 18 swimsuit had split at the seams.) When she was slim, she dreamed, she would be so happy.

When I met Penny she weighed eighteen stone, and she was really depressed. She had been promoted several times and although she was earning enough money to support herself, she was still saying that she planned to leave her husband, change jobs and begin swimming, when she got slim.

During her time in therapy Penny realized that she was using her weight problem as an excuse not to do the things she really wanted to. She was terrified to face up to Tom and tell him that she was leaving. She was scared of living alone, being alone. While she kept on thinking about how much weight she was going to lose, she did not have to face just how unhappy she really was.

Penny began with the least frightening of the three major things she was using her weight problem to put off. She went swimming. Because she was so anxious, she kept reciting the things we had rehearsed in her therapy sessions: 'I approve of myself, I love swimming, if anybody looks at me and notices how fat I am I will not shrivel into a ball nor will I die. If they notice me, I will not affect their lives, nor will they think of me for more than half a minute before they go on to their next thought. It is my own thoughts that make me so miserable. If anybody does make a comment about my weight

I will wonder what is wrong with them that makes them want to be cruel. I approve of myself. Going swimming is good for me, if I stay at home I will get miserable and eat. I approve of myself.'

And she did it – she walked from the changing-room to the pool, got in the pool and swam and swam, and loved it. She got out of the pool at the exit nearest the ladies' changing-room and charged in as fast as she could. But she did it, and she did it again, and again, until she went swimming without even thinking about what size she was.

In the ensuing months Penny consulted a lawyer, and after a stormy confrontation with Tom she moved out into a flat, which she shared with two other people. She is currently sending off job applications whenever she sees a job that she likes the sound of.

I wonder what things you are putting off because you feel you have to lose weight first. Buying new clothes? Having another baby? Changing your job or going back to college? Learning to dance or play tennis? Finding a new partner?

Life is happening now! If we keep putting off living until we are slim then we will stay stuck. The years are rolling on. Take those changes you keep putting on hold, take a deep breath and take the leap. Make them now!!!

9. I Am What I Weigh

During my first year in medical school I lost five stone using Dr Jack's diet. I bought him a gift and thanked him for all the help he had given me. Then exams came along and I began to put on weight. Well, Dr Diet had not taught me how to eat; he taught me how to diet. He didn't tell me that being on such a calorie-restricted diet would slow my metabolic rate down. He didn't even mention that because I had been overweight right through adolescence I might have difficulty with my sexuality.

He didn't warn me that in times of stress I would turn to food. He didn't tell me that only two out of 100 people succeed on diets.

He told me how to diet, and when I went back to see him after I had gained ten pounds he made it perfectly clear that it was all my fault, that I had once again failed. He told me I was 'naughty', and that I must go back on his diet and do it properly this time.

I easily agreed with him – I had been blaming myself for years. Every time I put on weight I felt as if I had failed. I forgot that I was just as unhappy when I was thin. My self-hatred grew and grew. I felt as if I was the problem. I was a bad person because I was fat, I was a bad person because I couldn't stick to a diet.

We make a decision about ourselves somehow, we decide that being fat is equal to being bad, so we hate ourselves for being fat. Then we diet, and even though diets don't work we blame ourselves for the failure, not the diet. Abuse is heaped upon abuse, and we hate ourselves even more.

Please don't hate yourself, you are the weight you are right now because of everything that has happened in your life. It is OK to forgive yourself, to reach out to yourself, to understand that over the years you have developed a problem with food, and that does not make you a bad person. Eventually you will come to understand why you reach for food when you are not hungry, and it is that understanding which will free you from your weight problem.

You are lovely and special whatever weight you are.

10. Who Is in Control?

Many people think that losing weight is all about self-control over one's appetite, over food. When we have periods of overeating we call it being out of control, and we are told that in order to lose weight we need to control the amount that we eat.

But when we follow a diet, and are told exactly what and how much to eat, the diet book, or club or programme becomes our master. We let people who don't know us tell us exactly what and how much to eat, even if it is food we do not like, at times when we are not hungry. I remember that when I was following the Weight Watchers programme I swallowed down the prescribed breakfast, every morning, without any enjoyment. Bran flakes with skimmed milk, or a boiled egg – food I didn't like, food I would not normally choose. After all, I was sticking to the diet. I gave up my power of choice in order to follow the programme. I ignored my own taste and appetite and forced down food I disliked because the programme told me to.

Diets encourage us to deny our hunger and follow other people's rules: no food after nine o'clock at night, ten glasses of water a day, no butter. We eat horrible combinations of food and dried-out slimming bars. We eat what the diet tells us, and when the diet is over we overeat because we want all the things that we were not allowed to eat when we were dieting. Who is really in control? Is this really self-control?

I have to live with myself for the rest of my life. I need to take back the control over my eating that I handed over to the diet doctors and clubs. I do not want to weigh and measure everything that I eat for ever and ever. I wish to decide what and how much to eat for myself. The choice is mine. If I am hungry for breakfast I will have some, if I am not hungry I won't have breakfast just because some expert tells me I must never skip breakfast. Either way the decision is mine, I am in control, I decide.

11. Is Fat Really Unhealthy?

Carmen told me about this typical conversation she had had with her mother, who had arrived for a visit:

Mother: I have heard about this fantastic new diet, Carmen. Instead of breakfast and lunch you buy this special powder in different flavours which you mix into a milkshake – they even have chocolate. Then you have a low-calorie supper. You can lose up to a pound every day.

Carmen, with a sigh: Yes.

Mother: Well, I thought you might like to try it. You really have gained a lot of weight lately.

Carmen: Mum, I wish you would leave me alone. I am comfortable about my weight. My whole life I have dieted and battled to be a size 12 and I will never be that. I am happy as I am right now. It is the first time for years that I have experienced peace with my eating, and that is because I gave up dieting.

Mother: But I am so worried, Carmen. I love you whatever size you are, but being fat is so unhealthy. All that extra weight is likely to cause you all sorts of health problems, and people who are fat are likely to die younger.

How many times have you heard people express that opinion? I know a lot of overweight people who fear going to their GP because even if their complaint has nothing to do with their weight, they feel sure that a comment will be made about it – and they are often right.

It is absurd to think that whether we are healthy or not depends on whether we are fat or slim. Health results from a combination of factors, including the nutritive value of everything that we drink and eat, and whether we use substances like drugs, cigarettes and alcohol. Our health also depends on how much exercise we take, where we live, what work we do, our family history and how stressful our lives are. Studies which look at only one major factor, like body weight, are too one-dimensional and will not give the complete picture.

The obvious question to ask is: what exactly are the health hazards of being overweight? At first glance the literature about the relationship between weight and health is confusing – no, it is more than confusing, it is like a war zone.

The words 'fat' and, especially, 'obesity' have very negative connotations in today's society. Obesity is the medical term used to describe the condition in which the body's fat stores become too large, and it is usually measured in terms of the relationship between the individual's height and weight. When a person is so large that his excess weight is causing serious health problems he is said to be morbidly obese.

But what are these demon fat stores that make us too large? Fat is often seen as treacherous, revolting, even cancer-like, as it attacks and crawls around our bodies. Actually, fatty tissue is an important natural part of our bodies. Women are built differently from men, and it is naturally occurring deposits of fat which give women their shape. Not only are these fat deposits important for women's figures, but the fatty tissue has an important reproductive and protective function. Fatty tissue is a store for oestrogen and the other sex hormones, and when the fat stores fall below a certain level, there is a corresponding drop in the level of these hormones. Oestrogen has an important protective effect against heart disease, high cholesterol and osteoporosis, and hormonal imbalance increases the risk of endometrial and ovarian cancer.

Women who are underweight, and women who diet and exercise to a unnatural leanness, have a 20 per cent chance of menstrual irregularities and infertility. If underweight women do manage to conceive they double their risk of having low-birth-weight babies.

Obesity has often been called a killer disease, but is this true? Numerous studies have been done to monitor people's weight, height and lifestyle from youth to death, in order to find out what they died from. The largest study was carried out on the population of Norway, where nearly two million participants were studied over ten years. The highest death rate occurred in those women who were *underweight*, and these women were twice as likely to die as women who were three or four stone heavier. The *lowest* mortality rate of all was found in women who were approximately 30 per cent overweight, but even those women who were morbidly obese had lower death rates than the underweight groups. For women there are in fact several health advantages to being fat, with reports of a lower incidence of certain cancers, osteoporosis, and some respiratory and infectious diseases.

Similar studies have shown the same pattern for men. Those who were underweight were much more likely to die prematurely than those who were normal weight or plump. But the distribution of body weight is particularly important for men, and it seems that those who develop a large stomach (beer belly) are at greater risk of heart conditions and blood sugar problems than their slim counterparts or those with fat distributed more evenly.

Another faulty assumption about weight and health comes from the numerous studies showing a correlation between obesity and medical conditions such as hypertension and diabetes. The word correlation here is the key. If somebody did a study which showed that of all the men who died of heart attacks in 1994, 78 per cent of them were married, we could then say that there is a correlation between people who are married and the occurrence of heart attacks. This would of course be grossly wrong because all the possible underlying factors would not have been taken into account. Even though many people who suffer heart attacks are overweight, there is no evidence to show that *just* being overweight is the cause. We would need to know if these men were smokers, if they exercised or not, what kind of lifestyle they had.

Health depends on a wide variety of factors. Fat deposits on the arteries and heart disease and high blood pressure occur in thin as well as fat people. There are many thin people who eat a high-fat diet and will have clogged arteries and heart disease,

while a fat person who eats more healthily will have much
clearer arteries and less risk of ill-health.

So, if you are healthy and overweight, there is no evidence to
show that the extra weight will cause ill-health. Smoking is much
more unhealthy than being overweight. Yo-yo dieting and crash
dieting are much more unhealthy than being overweight. However, if you are morbidly obese – can no longer weigh yourself
on normal bathroom scales – then there will be no way you can
avoid some ill-health because of this. If you already suffer from
the medical conditions of high blood pressure, diabetes, angina
and high cholesterol, and you are overweight, then losing weight
will help you control your disease.

12. Crash Diets Can Kill You

The damage that can be done to our bodies when we lose
weight too rapidly – especially on a very low-calorie diet –
is frightening. General medical opinion states that safe weight
loss should never be more than half a pound to a pound a
week. Losing weight too rapidly causes terrible stress on the
body. But there is a whole range of diets on the market which
are extremely low-calorie. Many consist of meal replacements
in liquid, powder or bar form.

The last diet I ever tried (and the most uncomfortable) was a
well-known liquid meal replacement diet which supplied a total
of 450 calories a day. The immediate side-effects of this diet were
actually listed on the packet: dizziness, nausea, constipation, bad
breath, headaches and dry skin. I felt really sick for a lot of the
time. My constant hunger made me really irritable – I shouted
at my boyfriend, especially when he was eating. I couldn't sleep
because I was so hungry. I felt awful!

I would have felt worse if I had known the long-term
side-effects of such a crash diet. When there is a sudden and
sharp decrease in the amount of calories you take in, your body

will switch to a lower metabolic rate. When you are not taking in enough energy your body provides you with the energy you need from your energy store. You may think that this would be your fat stores, but this is not so. There is not enough time for your body to mobilize your fat stores, so initially the sugar store in the liver is used up, and then the body begins to attack muscle tissue to provide energy. The problem is that the heart is also a muscle, and is not spared. If tissue from your heart is lost it can never be replaced.

As well as the potential heart problems caused by this loss of muscle tissue, very low-calorie diets can lead to loss of bone mineral, hair loss, depression and dehydration. The dehydration, combined with the low intake of calories, can cause an upset in the biochemical balance of the blood which in turn can cause cardiac arrhythmias and heart attacks. The low blood sugar levels which are induced on low-calorie diets will cause problems with concentration, low energy levels, markedly decreased sexual desire and depression. However, some crash dieters, and people who fast, can by contrast experience a feeling of euphoria due to the endorphins released by the brain. This in itself can be addictive, and can lead to too much weight loss, anorexia and all the physical effects of starvation.

Then let's look at what happens when you begin to eat normally again after the diet. First you will gain weight – 98 per cent of us will. And the weight gain is not the worst of it, because the muscle tissue which was lost on the diet is not replaced; rather, the extra weight gain is all fat. Also, when dieters regain weight after rapid loss their blood pressure rises to a higher level than before the diet, and it stays there – this is called a refeeding hypertension. The rapid weight gain is also associated with a higher cholesterol level, and can lead to the onset of diabetes and heart strain. You can imagine what happens if a person repeats this pattern over and over, crash diet, rapid weight gain, back on the crash diet: these problems can multiply. *People have died* as a result of the heart and blood pressure side-effects of yo-yo dieting and refeeding hypertension.

Crash dieting is *much* more unhealthy than being overweight.

13. Diets Can Lead to Eating Disorders

Research has shown that just *one* diet can lead to an obsession with food. What then is the result of years of dieting? If we continue to diet, our obsession with food and our weight will grow and grow.

Sandy had eaten a tuna roll for lunch. She had ordered the roll in an agony of indecision – when she walked into the sandwich shop she knew that what she really wanted was the salami and mortadella on an Italian roll, but she was too worried about all the fat in the meat and the cheese. The only low-calorie item she could see was her usual cottage cheese and salad roll, but she was tired of that. She remembered that when she was following Weight Watchers she was allowed tuna for lunch, and she remembered to have wholemeal instead of white. So she settled for tuna on a brown health roll. When she bit into the roll she realized that it was smothered in mayonnaise, and her heart sank as she imagined the mayonnaise turning into an instantaneous extra glob of fat on her thighs. She toyed with the idea of either scraping off the mayonnaise or ordering another roll, but all her indecision got swept up into a panic and she ended up eating the roll in huge gulps. As she ate a voice in her head was shouting: 'I shouldn't have this, I shouldn't be eating this.' But she did eat it, quickly, without enjoyment, and as soon as it was finished the critical voice continued to speak to her. 'You are so fat and you ate tuna *smothered in mayonnaise*. What is the matter with you, what is the matter with you? You will never get thin. Look at what you look like, the skirt you have on is a size 16!!! And it's cutting into your piles of revolting fat. You are a weak, despicable, horrible fat person.' The more this voice shouted at her, the worse Sandy felt, and eventually she just switched off from the voice, and from herself. She still had fifteen minutes of her lunch break left, so she stopped at the bakery and bought four chocolate doughnuts, and ate two on the way to the newsagent, where she bought three packets of crisps and a Mars bar. She took her pile of food into the office and hid it in her desk drawer, where it lasted for about half an hour because her hand kept snaking into the drawer and breaking off bits of food. She spent the rest of the afternoon daydreaming about what she could eat that night. She planned to make grilled chicken breast, but since she had blown it anyway, she decided that she would rather order a take-away curry . . . or a pizza . . . no, and a pizza, then she could have ice-cream for dessert . . . or she could make an instant pudding . . .

Jill was at home reading. All of a sudden images of the food from her fridge floated on to the pages of the book in front of her. She was not at all hungry but somehow a compelling force pulled her into the kitchen. She dipped her fingers into the leftover lasagne, then she finished off the potato salad, then she took a handful of biscuits back into the room with her to keep her company as she was reading. As she chewed the last biscuit she decided to drive to the petrol station for chocolate. 'I'm just going out to buy some milk,' she shouted to her husband, as she emptied the remains of the carton of milk into the sink. By the time she returned, all the chocolate she had bought was finished and she had begun to feel ill. That did not stop her – she put a frozen apple strudel into the microwave, but it took too damn long, so she took it out and ate it half frozen, and raw. By now she was really ill, ill enough to look in the rubbish bin for the hamburger her daughter had discarded at tea-time – and she ate that as well.

To a naturally slim person the behaviour of both Sandy and Jill is hard to understand. Yet I know that as you read their stories you may find their behaviour strangely familiar. Uncomfortably familiar. Both Sandy and Jill are compulsive eaters – they constantly think about how fat they are and how much weight they would like to lose, but they both constantly

eat when they are not hungry. Once they have eaten they give
themselves a real tongue lash if they feel they have eaten too
much.

I recently participated in a three-way debate, on radio, with
a representative from a well-known Scottish slimming club and
a nutritionist from Glasgow University. During the heated and
lively discussion about dieting, I mentioned that giving compulsive eaters a diet was like treating a patient who needed
antibiotics with strawberries. The lady from the slimming club
was astounded by my calling them compulsive eaters: 'But
Cherie, you cannot call people who come to us compulsive
eaters, we just take people who want to lose weight,' she said.
But I knew that most of the people who come to me also 'just
want to lose weight'. I also knew that these people had failed
at numerous diets, had despaired as the pounds they had fought
to lose crept back on. I knew that these people woke up thinking
about food and went to sleep worrying about their weight. Their
weight problem had travelled far beyond the point where a diet
would solve it. Their life had become a struggle, a daily battle
about food and eating and weight problems.

The lady from the slimming club continued. 'Come to us,' she
said. 'We will teach you to modify your eating habits. There are
special tricks you will learn, like using low-fat margarine instead
of butter, and Diet Coke instead of the regular sugared variety. If
you grill rather than fry your food you will be amazed how you
can cut down your calorie intake . . .' The programme hostess
expressed surprise, and asked her if she seriously thought that
most dieters did not know about Diet Coke and low-fat food.
'Of course they do not,' she replied. 'If people knew these things,
if they followed our advice, they would not always regain the
weight they had lost.'

I became angry, so angry I wanted to take the microphone
and twist it around her neck. Did she not hear what I heard?
Was she not aware of the hundreds of intelligent, articulate
people who know so much about nutrition and low-calorie
food that they could pass an exam on the subject? People

who nevertheless continuously battle and struggle with their eating?

Only the night before, Leonora had asked me if she was insane. 'I must be insane, Cherie, I want to be thin, I am desperate to be thin. I hate this fat on me, I hate it. I never look in mirrors if I can help it, but if I do I want to die; can this fat person be me? But when food is there and I am there I eat it. I am a logical thinking adult and I know that too much food makes me fat. But it is as if my brain does not make the connection between food and gaining weight. When food is there I just have to eat it.'

Eating disorder? Compulsive eater? I realize these are strong, perhaps shocking words. Many people, like the lady from the diet club, think that all compulsive eaters are enormously fat, weak-willed, despicable individuals. I know that is wrong. If your hand reaches for food when you are not hungry, if you have a constant desire for food, if the first thought that you have in the morning is food, and so is the last thought at night, if you want to eat when you are not hungry, if you continue to eat when you are full, if thoughts about food and eating and losing weight continuously creep into your mind, if you translate every feeling into a desire for food, then you have an eating disorder and that eating disorder is called compulsive eating.

Compulsive eating is an eating disorder because it is not natural or normal to spend every waking moment in a tug-of-war about whether we should or should not eat. It is horrible to spend our days and nights and lives struggling with food. Society has come to condone this behaviour as normal. It is not, it is self-destructive, energy-sapping and ultimately depressing.

Not all fat people are compulsive eaters, nor are all compulsive eaters fat. It is not dependent on how you look but on how you feel inside. Most compulsive eaters share an intense desire to be slim, and if that desire is coupled with a fear of being fat they sometimes keep themselves really thin by controlling every morsel of food that they eat. These people are also referred to as chronic dieters, and they are in as much pain as compulsive eaters. A compulsive eater may demolish a whole lemon meringue pie. The chronic dieter won't have any lemon meringue, but she will obsessively think about eating it. A chronic dieter spends as much thought energy on food as a compulsive eater – a thin person with a fat mind.

The compulsive eater is in a no-win position. One part is desperate to be thin, and the other part is desperate to eat. To eat or not to eat is the war raging within her – between meals, at mealtimes, in fact most of the time. No wonder it becomes an obsession.

We have all heard of the eating disorders highlighted by the media: anorexia nervosa and bulimia nervosa are outside the province of this book, and they can be life-threatening conditions. If you think you are anorexic or bulimic, I cannot urge you strongly enough to seek out specialist medical help. But anorexia nervosa (the condition of extreme weight loss where sufferers eat progressively less and less) and bulimia nervosa (the binge–purge disease where sufferers eat huge amounts and then try to get rid of what they have eaten by vomiting and laxative abuse) are both accepted by the medical profession as having part of their roots in dieting. But what about compulsive eating? TWENTY-FIVE PER CENT OF WOMEN ARE USUALLY ON A DIET AT ANY TIME, and 90 per cent of women will have dieted at some point in their lifetime. And we are all encouraged to keep on dieting in perpetuity, which increases the severity of our compulsive eating.

Compulsive eating comes in varying degrees of severity, depending on just how much thought energy is involved and on how exactly your overeating, or undereating and weight obsession affects the way you live your life. Only you can decide whether you are a compulsive eater or not. Throughout this book I will use the term compulsive eating to mean that you are constantly driven to eat when you are not hungry or that you deny yourself food when you are.

Whatever the degree, compulsive eating deserves our attention. We need to stop, analyse and give loving care and attention to our problem. For me, overcoming my compulsive eating, and the resultant self-understanding, was the most important thing I have ever done for myself.

14. The Diet Treadmill

Once upon a time there was a girl called Beth. She was a lovely girl, with a nice curvy figure. Beth, unfortunately, lived in a society which says that in order to be attractive you have to be thin, and once you are thin you will be happy. All Beth's friends and every magazine she reads tells her about dieting, tells her that the softness on her legs is called cellulite, and it will go if she eats no fat whatsoever. She hears words like 'thunder thighs', 'roly-poly', and because she does not look like the models she sees in her magazine Beth decides she had better try a diet, 'just to see what happens'. She finds the diet quite easy, and she loses five pounds. She hauls out the dress she wore to her eighteenth birthday party and is thrilled when she easily zips into it. She begins to eat again and just a few weeks later she is dismayed to find that she has gained six pounds. Her friend is on a meal replacement diet and she decides to try that for a few weeks. She loses weight, but then she gains it, then loses again, then she gains. A few years later she is totally obsessed with food and her weight; she cannot stop at one chocolate, she binges, then she undereats. Her metabolic rate is slowed down. Her self-esteem is wrapped up in her weight. Her conversation is all about weight. She longs for those days when she used to eat what she wanted. She wonders why she thought she was fat when she was five pounds overweight. She keeps on looking for a new diet.

During my workshop I give participants this questionnaire to fill in. Do try it: it will give you the opportunity to see exactly what has happened to you over the years of dieting:

1. List the diets you have been on in the past. For each one, state if you reached your goal weight and, if so, for how long you were able to maintain it.
2. Do you think that the next diet you go on will be the one that works for ever?
3. When did you go on your first diet?
4. What weight were you when you began dieting?
5. What weight are you now?
6. Consider your answers to questions 4 and 5. Has dieting been successful for you in the long term?
7. Why do you keep on dieting if it has not been successful for you in the past?

We need to eat in order to stay alive; if we stop eating we will die. Food is an integral part of our lives – we need to shop for food, make lunch for our children, and have dinner parties with friends. TV adverts bombard us with rivers of chocolate and Chicken McNuggets. We are surrounded by food everywhere, fast food in the streets, sweets at every service station, pizza delivered to our door. In the midst of all this food we go on a diet. We restrict ourselves, we watch and measure how much we eat. We wake up every morning and tell ourselves we have to live on liquid shakes and Diet Coke. Don't eat this, measure that. No salad dressing, no butter. Handcuffs please, gag over mouth please. Life is filled with chores and duties, things we have to do, and then we put ourselves into diet prison. This person is innocent, but heaven forbid she should know this. Sentence her to diet jail and make sure that she stays there. For ever.

The psychologist B. F. Skinner studied how and why human beings behave the way they do. He and a group of other researchers carried out a very interesting experiment. They taught a group of rats and a group of people to run a maze. Every time the rats had successfully completed their maze they were given a piece of cheese as a reward for doing so, and each time the humans had completed their maze their reward was $10. The researchers allowed this to continue for a while, then they stopped giving the rewards. So the rats completed the maze and there was no cheese, the people completed their maze and there was no money. Guess what happened?

After the rats had run the maze several times without getting any reward, they lost interest, and stopped doing it. The people didn't. They kept on, running the maze over and over again. The result was failure each and every time, but somehow they would not give up.

If we have been dieting for years and years then we are like those people who kept on running the maze long after the $10 reward had stopped. We are not only wasting time and energy, we are also disappointing ourselves over and over again.

So we run on round, and round the treadmill ... which leads us nowhere. Don't do it. Explain to your children why they shouldn't do it either. Please don't diet ever again.

I have shown you all the different and varied ways that dieting can be harmful, and I hope that you are now firmly convinced that dieting is not the solution, it is the problem. I can hear your next question: 'Well, Cherie, if diets don't work, what does?' In the next chapter I will start to answer that question, and show you how to live not only without dieting, but better, more healthily, and at the weight you are meant to be.

2

Eating Like a Naturally Slim Person

'When I gave up dieting I was terrified. Even though the diet–binge existence I was living was horrible it was familiar, and to lose it was like losing a friend. What would I do when I no longer had a diet to start on Monday? How would I live?'

IRENE — WEIGH AHEAD COURSE, SEPTEMBER 1993

'Food is an important part of a balanced diet.'

FRAN LIEBOWITZ

My friend Jeremy showed me a book called 'Your Baby's First Year', which his mother had proudly filled in sixty-one years ago. I got a sense of its age from the yellowing pages and the old-fashioned script. Just under the heading in the section called 'Feeding', Jeremy's mother had written: 'From the beginning

THE DESTRUCTIVE DIET CYCLE

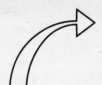

I begin a new diet.

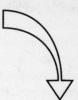

I feel strong and in control and weight loss begins.

As the diet progresses I begin to feel hungry and deprived. Inevitably I break the diet.

I eat, overeat and binge.

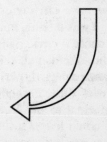

I regain the weight I have lost plus some extra pounds.

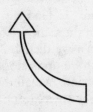

I feel fat, feel I have failed, and I am filled with self-loathing.

I continue to binge and overeat; in the moment of eating food makes me feel better.

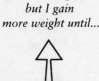

I hate being fat but I gain more weight until...

Jeremy was fed four-hourly with no feeds at night.' My heart grew cold as I read it, and I wanted to hug him to try and make better what had happened all those years ago. How can you not give a baby food at night? Surely he screamed and kicked and asked for food, again and again?

The bold handwriting clearly showed that a battle had been fought and won: 'From the beginning . . . no feeds at night' — between those lines I read another story: from the beginning, I taught Jeremy to deny his hunger at night. I thought it was the right and proper thing to do, to ignore his cries for food in the night, and anyway he eventually got so exhausted he stopped crying and slept through.

Jeremy never allows himself to get hungry now. He consistently overeats and often eats long before he becomes hungry. He hates being overweight, but hunger is terrifying for him. Hunger makes him feel as if he is alone and helpless in a cold, dark night.

Thank goodness, the idea of feeding babies by the clock like Jeremy's mother did has gone out of fashion. Over the last four decades the experts have realized that the best way to feed a baby is on demand. There is no need to impose any restrictions or schedules on a baby's feeding pattern. When a baby is hungry he will cry for food, and when that baby has eaten enough he will close his mouth and lose interest. We are all born with the ability to eat just enough, to eat exactly what our body needs. Our brain controls the whole system simply and effectively. We know we need to eat, because we get hungry; and when we have eaten enough the hunger goes away.

When I was dieting, hunger was my enemy, and in my student years I chose a circle of friends who ate in the same crazy way that I did. We dieted, then we binged, then we dieted. A very important part of our friendship was that we understood and shared each other's weight and food obsession. We all thought it was normal to live like that, and it never entered our heads that we could live in a different way.

During our fourth year at medical school we worked in

pairs as we rotated through the surgical, medical, obstetrical and paediatric teaching wards. I spent a lot of time with my partner, Clive, and the contrast in our eating patterns was easily seen. If I was dieting I would skip breakfast, eat an apple for lunch and choose the lowest-calorie items I could find in the hospital canteen at dinner. Clive always ate porridge for breakfast, a two-course lunch and a huge plate of dinner. In addition he would often fill his plate with sandwiches or biscuits at each tea-break. The first few days I spent with Clive, I thought he was on a binge, but to my amazement he ate like that most days.

I knew the calorific value of every single morsel I ate. Clive never gave a thought to calories or food quantities. He never deprived himself of food, nor did he think about eating when he was not hungry. I did, all the time. Clive loved good food and he would often make a detour to buy his favourite food treat. I ate my favourite food sneakily, only on binge days. The only time there was a change in Clive's eating pattern was when he was anxious or upset – at exam time, or when he had split up with his girlfriend. Then he hardly ate at all, he just couldn't. If I was upset or angry or anxious I ate continuously. My weight fluctuated wildly and Clive's weight always stayed the same.

It was only when I read Bob Schwartz's book *Diets Don't Work* that I found an explanation for Clive's eating pattern. He was, and is, a naturally slim person, and he continued to demand feed himself as he grew into adulthood. Instead of watching with envy as Clive piled up his plate, I should have been asking him these questions: 'How do you know you need to eat? Why did you have three sandwiches on Tuesday, and none on Wednesday? Why is food and eating not an issue for you?' Clive would have been able to answer those questions better than any diet expert because he was a naturally slim person. He intuitively knew how to eat. He never dieted, and never lost touch with his body hunger.

For us the years of dieting made us lose touch with the eating wisdom that we were born with. Instead of eating when we were hungry, we imposed all sorts of restrictions on ourselves. We learnt not to mix certain foods, we learnt to eat rice cakes when we craved bread and butter. We were told not to eat after nine o'clock. We ate no fat because Rosemary Conley said we shouldn't, we ate fruit because Judy Mazel said we should, and we ate protein when the Scarsdale diet was in fashion.

How can we possibly tell if we are hungry? We have followed so many diet rules and regulations that we have lost touch with our bodies. Not only have we forgotten that the only time to eat is when we are really hungry, but we have forgotten *what real hunger is*.

This becomes obvious in my talks and trainings, from the questions that I get asked. How much should I eat? How many glasses of water should I drink each day? What am I allowed? Can I mix potato with fish? Grown adults ask these questions: they have become childlike. They have become so used to being told what to eat that they don't know what they want, or what their body needs.

The answer I give is always the same. Eat like naturally slim people. Eat when you are hungry, eat exactly what you are hungry for, and stop eating when you are satisfied. 'But how will I lose weight?' they ask. 'How will I know when I am hungry?'

To a chronic dieter the thought of living in total freedom with food is a completely alien concept. When we diet we are undereating, and when we binge we are overeating. Living this way brings utter chaos and confusion into our lives. We need to learn to live and eat without overeating, and without undereating. Only then can we begin to solve our weight problem. Only then can we be free.

I have written this book to provide support for you as you go through this change from abnormal to normal eating. There is magic, but there is also hard work. The magic is that you can reconnect with the naturally slim person within you. The hard work is that you have to learn how to say no to food that you want when you are not hungry. It took years of diet restrictions before you were placed in this food prison with the door so firmly shut. Step by step we need to travel on a journey of change. We unlock the prison door when we stop dieting, but in order to actually leave our cell, we have some important work to do: We need to look at what happened in our past, to unravel exactly how we developed our weight problem in the first instance.

The first step, then, is to give up all forms of dieting: that means any food or eating prescriptions or meal plan of any sort. Pack away your food-measuring scales. Give away your diet books, calorie counters, and lists of hidden fat content in food. Avoid the diet section in magazines and throw away all your artificial sweeteners, diet bars, meal replacement powders, crispbreads and rice cakes – unless you really like any of these foods. Stop talking about dieting and stop thinking about dieting. Don't weigh or measure yourself either. Weighing yourself once, twice or thirty times a day just increases the obsession. If you cannot bring yourself to throw away your scales you may need to wean yourself off gradually. Stop weighing yourself daily – limit it to once a week, then once a fortnight, then once a month, then not at all. It's not how much you weigh that counts but how you feel inside.

When you give up dieting you can begin to teach yourself to eat, like a naturally slim person. There are four basic principles involved.

1. Naturally slim people only eat when they are hungry.
2. Naturally slim people eat exactly what they feel like eating, what they are hungry for.
3. Naturally slim people enjoy their food and focus attention on what they are eating.
4. Naturally slim people stop eating when they are satisfied, when their bodies signal to them they have had enough.

For the rest of this chapter I will discuss these four basic principles in more detail.

1. Eating When You Are Hungry

The memory of a child who was in the same hospital as my son Alan keeps coming back to me. She was chronically ill with cystic fibrosis and had been admitted to hospital because, as she put it: 'I don't want to eat any more.' At mealtimes, when the other children were tucking in to their lunch, she sat with her plate of food and looked at it. The nurses tried their best and sat with her, negotiating for ten minutes before she would eat one cold chip. The food held absolutely no interest for her. When she did put anything in her mouth she could barely chew it, and when she tried to swallow it was as if the food would stick in her painfully thin throat. She was starving but she had totally lost her appetite. She no longer got hungry because she no longer wanted to live. How much she weighed had absolutely nothing to do with it. She could not eat and feed herself life-giving energy because she did not want energy. Her will to live and with it her appetite had slipped away from her.

Our hunger is a message from our bodies that we need to eat to give ourselves nourishing, life-giving energy. When I was dieting I lived my life cursing my hunger; now I celebrate feeling hungry. My hunger means I am alive, and I want to stay alive. I enjoy being hungry and I enjoy eating when I am hungry.

When we were babies and we got fed when we were hungry it must have been a perfectly satisfying experience. If, however, we got fed when we were tired or cold, then very early on we learned to eat as a response to tiredness and coldness. We learned to answer needs other than hunger with food. So we got confused. Dieting further confused us because we then started to ignore our hunger because of a programme that we were following. This I am sure is the reason why so many of my course participants complain that they don't know if they are hungry or not.

Getting in Touch with Your Hunger

We can rectify this confusion by getting back in touch with our hunger, our body hunger. We are all different, so the way we receive our hunger signal will be different. Some of us may feel hunger in our stomach, while others may feel it in their throat, or head. We will feel a rumbling or a grumbling or a gnawing signal *somewhere in our bodies*. This is body hunger. We all know the other kind of hunger, emotional hunger, wanting to eat because the food is there, or because the diet starts tomorrow, or because we don't know what to do with ourselves if we don't eat something. This is mouth hunger.

I used to feel as if I was hungry all the time, but I had forgotten the difference between wanting to eat because I was bored, lonely and depressed, and wanting to eat for genuine stomach hunger. For years I had let diet clubs and doctors tell me how and when to eat. I had to learn to take back the control over my own eating. I had to learn to trust myself enough to listen to the signals from my body.

When I am moderately hungry, I feel an empty, lightly burning sensation midway down my chest. As my hunger increases, the burning changes to a hollow feeling which extends into my stomach. Sometimes my hunger causes a feeling of slight nausea, and if I am too hungry I feel irritated and light-headed.

We have to throw away all our previous habits and beliefs and begin to experiment with eating in a totally new way. Disregard the usual routine of breakfast, lunch and dinner. In the morning, when you wake up, ask yourself, am I hungry? If you are, have breakfast. If you are not hungry, wait until you are hungry. Each day may be different – some days I am hungry at lunch-time, and on other days I am hungry for six small meals throughout the day. I suggest that you spend the next few months really getting to know yourself and your hunger patterns.

The Hunger Day

Before you begin, do try to discover exactly how you experience hunger. We all feel our hunger in different ways, so it really helps to do the following exercise, which we call the Hunger

Day. This is an experiment to identify how and when you feel physical hunger.

Choose a day when you have time and space to pay attention to yourself. When you wake up in the morning ask yourself: Am I hungry? If you think you are hungry, eat something small like a slice of toast. If you are not hungry, go and do something else, and wait for the hunger to come. Notice how you feel about skipping breakfast. You can keep reassuring yourself that this is not a diet, it is an experiment to identify how your body signals real hunger to you. Either way, whether you have breakfast or not, don't eat again until you are ravenously hungry. Closely observe yourself this day, notice how your body signals hunger to you, and write down how you feel at each stage. Perhaps you may feel mild hunger as a burning sensation, or an empty space somewhere in your body. As your hunger intensifies you may get a slight headache, or even a severe one. Try to identify *where* in your body you feel hunger at each stage. In your head? Your mouth? Your throat, chest, stomach, abdomen? Stay with your hunger, recording it as you go along, until you have reached a point when you are ravenously hungry. When you have reached that point, the experiment has been completed, and you can eat normally again. Drink normally throughout the day, however, whenever you are thirsty.

At the end of your Hunger Day, you should have a written record of what 'body hunger' feels like for you, from mild hunger through to ravenous hunger.

Barbara reported this to the group after her Hunger Day: 'I discovered that when I am mildly hungry, I feel a tingling in my mouth and throat. When I get to be moderately hungry, I feel a hollowness in my chest, and when I am really ravenous, I feel lightheaded, almost dizzy, and my stomach really rumbles out loud!'

Using a Hunger Gauge to Stop When Enough Is Enough

Once you are comfortable that you have identified your hunger, you need to pinpoint how your body signals it is satisfied. The object of eating when you are hungry is not to eat until you are full to bursting, it is to eat until you have had just enough. You will find it helpful to measure how hungry you are on a hunger gauge with a scale from zero to eight:

0 Desperately hungry. Starving and shaky.
1 Ravenously hungry. A small amount of food will not satisfy this hunger, and once you start eating it will be difficult to stop.
2 Very hungry. There is still a danger of overeating to compensate.
3 Moderately hungry. This is the ideal time to eat.
4 Mildly hungry. Only a few more bites needed to be satisfied.
5 Satisfied. Have eaten just enough.
6 Full. Have eaten a little too much.
7 Very full. Ignored the signal to stop eating and just kept on going. Feel really uncomfortable.
8 Overfull. So full that you could burst, feel real pain.

There are two important reasons for using the hunger gauge: first of all, it will help you learn to eat when you are hungry. Only dieters ignore their hunger. When your hunger reaches level 3, moderate hunger, it is the ideal time for you to eat. As soon as you feel the body signal that you know for you means level 3, eat something.

During the Hunger Day exercise I recommended that you allow yourself to get ravenously hungry, but it was only for that one day. Ravenous hunger has a life all of its own; enough food does not seem to be enough and we end up eating until we are overfull. Keep in touch with your hunger signals during the day, and demand feed yourself as soon as you are moderately hungry.

If you regularly feed yourself when you are moderately hungry, you will begin to trust your appetite again. This means that the need to overeat, or to eat before you get hungry, will dwindle.

The second reason to use the hunger gauge is to learn to stop when you are satisfied. This means stopping at level 5, when you are just satisfied. Initially you may continue to eat until level 6 or 7, but practice makes a huge difference.

Every time you want to eat, the first thing to ask yourself is: AM I HUNGRY? If the answer is yes, that is when to eat, because your body is signalling for food. You may get hungry every few hours, or only twice a day. Whatever spontaneous pattern emerges for you is the one to follow.

We really need to make a commitment to eating only when we are hungry. This may take some adjustment to one's life: for some it will be surprisingly complicated. I am lucky because I work at home and can easily eat whenever I am hungry, but for many of my course participants it is much more difficult, because their work is inflexible as regards meal-times, or because they are constrained by the need to cook for and feed a family. Whenever I speak to a group about eating when you are hungry there is immediately an uproar of questions.

You say disregard breakfast, lunch and dinner; but all the diets I've been on tell me it's very bad to skip meals.
Imagine if we lived in a society that had decided we should have five meals a day, or two, or ten? Then like robots we would all follow this tradition. Breakfast, lunch and supper are artificial creations, but they are so widely accepted that we rarely question them. The whole idea of eating like a naturally slim person means eating when you are hungry. Only then. Possibly the idea of breakfast, lunch and dinner were created because that is when most people do get hungry, but as you reconnect with your body, with your natural rhythms of hunger and eating, you need to step aside from traditional dictates. If you happen to get hungry at traditional meal-times, then by all means eat at those times. But what if you are not hungry at lunch-time? We want to stop all automatic eating. Think of animals in the wild. They are totally in tune with their bodies; they eat when they are hungry and sleep when they are tired. They have no need for clocks, or

alarm clocks, or fixed meal-times. I have never seen or heard of a fat wild animal – only domestic ones. We have an animal rhythm inside each and every one of us, and we need to tune into this. Our hunger will be different some days from others, and only by being in tune with ourselves can we respond to this difference. Nobody can tell you when you are hungry; only you will know, and you know because your body tells you. I know that I can trust my body to send me a hunger signal when I need to eat; trust yourself, and let your body hunger guide you.

You may have to warn your family or the people you are living with, and explain to them what you plan to achieve. Tell them that you may be eating breakfast at eleven and dinner at four; but explain that you are doing that in order to get back into your naturally slim eating rhythm that you have lost during years of dieting and compulsive eating.

What if I find I am hungry all the time?

The minute I suggest to you that you stop dieting, memories of all the previous occasions when you stopped dieting are going to surface. In your past, the end of a diet usually meant the start of a binge. Eating when you are hungry is a totally new way of living – it is not dieting, and it is not bingeing. It is eating when you are hungry. Not undereating followed by overeating, just eating. Eating normally and with enjoyment, because eating is part of being alive. If you learn to listen to your body hunger signals, and if you learn to trust and follow those signals, you will eat, and not overeat, and your weight will go to the level that it is meant to be at.

If you are eating when you are hungry and stopping when you are satisfied, there is no way that you can be body hungry all the time. Feeling hungry all the time is usually emotional hunger, not body hunger. If you find yourself eating all day, or wanting to eat an hour after a substantial meal, then you are looking to food to answer a need which is *not hunger*. The whole of the next chapter is devoted to this important issue.

Suppose I NEVER get hungry?

This is a very important question. It is a total misconception that overweight people never get hungry. Of course they do. We all need energy to walk, talk, breathe and stay alive, no matter what weight we are. You will get hungry, I promise you. I have found that many course participants find that they do not need much food in the first few weeks and months, but this is only while their body is burning their excess fat stores. As they reach the weight they are meant to be, their hunger increases. In the meantime I always tell them to trust their body to guide them.

What do I do about my family?

There is a long-standing tradition about family mealtimes. For many of us it is the only time when the whole family gets together. It is a time to sit down around a table and (ideally) talk and listen and catch up on each other's day: it is also a time when we eat. Of course, if you are hungry at the family mealtime, then eat and enjoy what you are eating. But many of the people at my workshops complain that they are not always hungry at the same time as the rest of the family. If you are not hungry, the companionship you seek from your partner or family, and the companionship they look to you for, is not dependent on you actually eating: it is supplied by your sitting down with them and listening to them. If you are not hungry and you still eat, there is a good chance that you will begin to feel so bad and guilty that you may withdraw emotionally from the people sitting around you, spoiling the togetherness you are all seeking. Better to sit and talk and listen without eating, explain that you are not hungry and put a plate aside for yourself for later.

Carol has four children – two teenagers, an eight-year-old daughter and a four-year-old son. She used to insist on the whole family sitting down to a meal as soon as her husband came home. She would spend the previous hour cooking, screaming at the teenagers not to eat Pop Tarts because it would ruin their dinner. Her younger son and daughter would be scuffling around her, wanting her attention, and she would nibble continuously as she cooked. After she had learned about eating when you are hungry, she decided to let the whole family try it. Everybody contributed to the shopping list and had their own favourite foods available. Carol would prepare a meal, and the whole family would sit down together. Those who were hungry would eat, and those who were not hungry would wait and have something later. Carol says that for the first time in sixteen years she actually relaxes at dinner-time. She talks to her children and does not continuously berate them for eating or not eating.

If I eat when I am hungry how can I possibly lose weight?

It is not eating that makes us gain weight, it is overeating. As you learn to eat only when you are hungry, and stop overeating, you will lose weight. But it will take time. Eventually, your weight will naturally stabilize at what it is meant to be.

I believe that our bodies all have a natural setpoint weight – that is, a normal weight that is programmed into our genes for maximum energy and fitness. Through the years of unnatural eating, of dieting and bingeing, our weight has fluctuated so much that we have completely lost sight of what our setpoint weight is. Our bodies know. Left to its own devices, your body will want to go back to the weight it is meant to be. Our bodies want to be light and energetic, not heavy and tired. So in order for your body to go back to its natural setpoint, it will give you hunger signals accordingly. How do we lose weight? If you eat only when you are hungry, your body will use the excess fat stores, and only ask for food when you need energy which it cannot immediately provide from our fat stores. This will take time. But you deserve to give yourself every minute of the time it takes.

What do I do at dinner parties?

We live in an age where socializing is usually done around food. We arrange to meet our friends for coffee or lunch, or we are invited over for dinner. The host or hostess at a dinner party will have spent hours preparing the meal and will expect their guests to eat with relish most of what is served to them. That person wants to be acknowledged for the time and trouble it has taken for them to cook the meal. Thank you, that must have taken ages, the food was absolutely wonderful, would you give me the recipe please?

Unfortunately we cannot arrange our hunger for our hosts, neither can we choose exactly what to eat. Naturally slim people often overeat at dinner parties and it is no big deal – without even thinking about it they will eat a bit less the next day. Overeating at one dinner party will not make you fat.

In my groups we brainstormed for dinner party solutions and here is what we came up with:

- If you know you are going to a dinner party, save your hunger during that day. What I mean is, when you are moderately hungry eat something small, like a piece of fruit or a small sandwich. Don't allow yourself to get too hungry, but it is OK to eat less than you usually do if you know you are going to have a big meal at night. A naturally slim person won't have a big lunch if she knows she is going out to an enormous meal later.
- Pace yourself throughout the meal: if there are going to be a number of courses eat a moderate amount of each course. Try saying, 'Thank you, this is delicious but I want to leave room for dessert.'
- If the hostess is a good friend, explain about this programme.
- When you are being served, ask for a small portion.
- Eat slowly.
- Don't worry that your host or hostess's feelings will be hurt if you do not eat with gusto and scrape your plate clean. Say what you have often heard naturally slim people say: 'This is absolutely delicious, but I cannot eat another mouthful because I am so full.' Ask for a recipe, or you could do

what Marion did at a dinner party. After the starters and main course she was feeling full. Her hostess brought out the dessert and she groaned. Trifle, her favourite. Marion had three choices: she could have one or two bites of the trifle, now, for the taste, or she could have a whole bowlful and suffer the consequences (feeling uncomfortable and full), or she could ask if she could take some home. Her hostess was delighted to give her a bowlful to take home, and that way Marion was able to say no to the trifle and not feel deprived, because she knew she could have some the next day when she was hungry, while her hostess was flattered rather than offended. You can do the same thing in a restaurant: ask for a doggy bag if you are satisfied, but unhappy about leaving food on your plate.

- Be careful about drinking too much alcohol, because when we are drunk we tend to throw caution to the winds and overeat.
- If you try but fail to avoid overeating, be very firm with yourself and say stop. Stop now. Don't slip back into that old diet mentality that says I've blown it anyway, so I may as well binge, but at the same time try and be kind and patient with yourself too. Remember to reassure yourself that you can eat again as soon as you are hungry, tomorrow.
- Stop thinking about the food, the portions, how much food you have eaten, and participate in the conversation instead.
- Enjoy yourself!!

May learned a very important lesson when she went to a dinner party at her friend's house. On the way over in the car she worked out that all she had left of her daily quota was 400 calories. She decided that she would allow herself one glass of wine and stick to low-fat food. May arrived, hung up her coat, and the loneliness that she was so used to descended upon her as she looked into the room, filled with several seemingly happy, chatting couples. She noticed that three of the women were wearing slinky party dresses, and she felt frumpy in her leggings and dark jumper. She was seated next to a friendly man at the dinner table. He said his name was Doug, and May found him really easy to talk to. While he was talking to the person on the other side the first course arrived. May began to worry about eating and not eating and how fat she was, so when Doug tried to resume a conversation with her she was distant and unfriendly. She continued to worry about fat content, and whether she was eating too much. After dinner her friend Sally, the hostess, came to look for her: 'What did you do to Doug? He said he was really enjoying talking to you and then you cut him dead.' May didn't answer — she had been so busy hiding herself away in her feelings of fatness and controlling her food intake that she had forgotten all about Doug. She took a deep breath and went over to talk to him. As they joked and flirted she forgot about her diet and her weight. At one point she looked over to the dinner table where she had spent the first half of the evening and realized that she had learnt a valuable lesson. Her companion for dinner had been her weight problem. Her loneliness was self-inflicted.

Why do I feel so scared at the thought of waiting to eat until I'm hungry?

Penny flopped gratefully into her allocated seat on the aeroplane. She and her friend Gill were going to Spain for a two-week holiday. Penny's day had been very busy as she rushed around packing and making all the last-minute preparations for her trip.

Penny and Gill groaned as the captain announced that their take-off time would be delayed — they were currently in a queue of aircraft waiting to take their turn on the runway. Penny was really hungry, and she was not happy at the thought that they would only get something to eat when they were up in the air. She began to feel anxious, slightly panicky. She could not concentrate on the magazine she had brought to read, nor was she interested in talking to Gill about all the things they were going to do on their holiday. She wanted food, and she wanted it *now*.

At long last the plane took off, but Penny's agitation began
to rise as the various cabin crew introduced themselves. She kept
craning around to see if the hostess with the food trolley was
anywhere near by. Her hunger and need for food were making
her so frantic that she was even close to tears. In the midst of
all this, Gill looked up from her book and said that she was so
hungry she could eat a horse – and then looked down at her
book again, as she continued to read. Even through her mounting panic Penny noticed that Gill had said she was ravenously
hungry and then had gone back to *reading*. Penny asked Gill if
she really meant what she had said about being hungry. 'Yes,'
Gill replied; and Penny realized that there was a huge difference
in the way they reacted to their hunger. When Penny was hungry the hunger became a driving force. It overrode most other
thoughts and feelings. Gill did not understand this – to her,
hunger was much less charged. She was hungry now, but there
was no food available, and although she was uncomfortable she
did not feel agitated, or frantic, and she was perfectly happy to
wait until there was some food.

I suppose you have guessed that Gill is a naturally slim
person. Penny, on the other hand, had been on the diet cycle
for years. The more she had deprived herself, the more food
had come to dominate her life. Food had come to symbolize
comfort, a friend when she was lonely, a soothing balm when
she was in pain. Of course she felt frightened when she was
hungry, it threatened the very core of everything she found safe
and comfortable.

It was only on that plane journey, when she saw how her
reaction to hunger was so different to Gill's, that she gained
the insight that hunger was frightening for her. She went to see
a therapist and together they worked out ways to help Penny
comfort and look after herself in other ways besides food.

It is worthwhile investigating how you were fed as a baby.
If, like Jeremy, you were deprived of food as a child, it will
help to explain why hunger scares you so much. Another
reason you may fear hunger may reach even further back.

During the Second World War my father was a prisoner of war in Italy for three years, and lost forty pounds in weight in that time. Hunger was a constant companion for him during those years, as he and his fellow prisoners were never given enough food to eat. After he got back from the war he would never allow himself to get hungry – it reminded him too much of those horrible, life-threatening years. Years later I was fascinated to read that children of parents who have suffered real starvation often show signs of having inherited the tremendous feelings of anxiety which their parents felt about hunger. The children had also learned to associate hunger with anxiety. Besides the years of diet deprivation, this helped to explain to me why I get frantic when I am hungry.

Take a minute now, and think about how you feel about being hungry. Think back on the last time you were really hungry and food was not close at hand. Once you have thought of your example, close your eyes, lie back, and imagine yourself back in that situation. How did you feel? What happened as the hunger intensified? Were you anxious? Afraid? Panicky? Was there a difference between the way you reacted and the way your companions did?

We can never make up for the years we sat starving while everybody ate. We cannot make up for the famine that we, or our parents, may have lived through in the war years. Those years are gone, they will not come back. The only thing that will come back if we stuff ourselves to compensate for former famine is extra weight. If you suffered deprivation during wartime rationing, then next time you are in a supermarket, have a good look around, and see just how much food there is available – there is no shortage of food now. You can never make up for undereating yesterday by overeating today. And you cannot compensate for dieting tomorrow by overeating today. Reassure yourself every day that there is plenty of food around. You need not fear hunger because you are never going to starve again.

I am terrified to leave the house without eating. What if I am hungry later?

If hunger terrifies you, there is a danger that you will eat when you are not hungry, just in case you get hungry later.

Karen always had a late evening meal and consequently was never hungry in the morning. When she began following this programme she realized that the two slices of toast she ate every morning were just a habit. She decided that she would skip breakfast, but to her own surprise this made her feel anxious. 'I felt so awkward leaving for work without breakfast,' she said. 'I was worried — what if I became hungry later?' Karen sells cosmetics and travels about in her car. To solve her problem she decided that she would take a sandwich with her so that she could eat it when she became hungry. That is what a naturally slim person would do. Naturally slim people rarely eat when they are not hungry, but they do arrange food for when they are hungry.

If you are committed to eating when you are hungry, but you do not always have instant access to the foods you might want, it is a good idea to take an emergency food pack with you wherever you go. I always have some fruit and a sesame snap in my bag. I have also been known to pack a muffin or scone or whatever my favourite food of the moment is. I have made a promise to myself that I will eat whenever I am moderately hungry, so I need to carry food around with me wherever I go.

Often, when I suggest this, people in my group say that if there is food around, they are likely to reach for it when they are not hungry. If in the initial stages of this programme you find that you cannot have the food with you because you will eat it whether you are hungry or not, put it somewhere where you cannot reach for it automatically: lock the food in the trunk of your car or get a lunch box on which you have written: 'Am I hungry? This food is for hunger only.' As you become more secure and comfortable about having food about, you will find that you are able to carry food without being tempted by it, and that you are even able to throw it away if you don't eat it. (Yes, really, I do that all the time.)

When I am at work how can I eat when I am hungry?
If you are not hungry at lunch, or at tea-break, I suggest you keep a sandwich in your desk drawer to eat later. If you are not allowed to eat at your desk you can experiment with regulating your hunger. If you want to be hungry at lunchtime you can try a smaller breakfast, or an earlier tea-break. Lunchtime at work happens five days a week, so it is worthwhile spending some time sorting out your hunger pattern.

I know that you can come up with a hundred different situations in which you will have to eat when you are not hungry, or when you cannot eat when you are. An occasional meal when you are not hungry is not going to blow the whole programme. But if you want to, I mean *really* want to eat only when you are hungry, then you should make a commitment to do so.

I believe that we are all born with the ability to eat normally, and no matter how long we have been on the diet–binge cycle, we still have the instinctive expertise of that naturally slim person within us. I trust you. I trust you to be able to rediscover the naturally slim person within you. I trust you to trust yourself.

2. Eating What You Really Want

Finding Out What Foods You Are Hungry For

A while ago I was on my way home from a trip to Edinburgh and I began to get hungry. I asked myself what I was hungry for and images of sticky toffee pudding came up. I stopped at Marks & Spencer and bought a huge pudding, but as I put the shopping into my car I started to criticize myself. 'You have not had anything nutritious the whole day, you can't fill up on white flour, butter and sugar.' When I got home I put the sticky toffee pudding into the fridge and decided to have a tuna salad.

I made a huge healthy salad and chopped onions into the tuna, and then sat and looked at it. I wanted sticky toffee pudding, with custard. I had to make a decision. I could wade through the salad and then spend the evening feeling unsatisfied. I knew that in the past, when I had had a meal which consisted of food I did not really want, I would spend the evening wandering back and forth to the kitchen − for nuts and raisins and then a few minutes later for carrots. So many times before have I ended up at midnight feeling uncomfortable, full and still unsatisfied. A few days later, or even the next day, I would end up giving in to my craving and bingeing on sticky toffee pudding.

I put the salad away, ate some pudding, thoroughly enjoyed it, curled up with my book and did not think about food for the rest of the evening.

Naturally slim people ask their bodies what they feel like eating and that is what guides them to choose. When a naturally slim person feels like eating pizza she eats pizza. When a habitual dieter feels like eating pizza, she eats a tomato and then a crispbread. Then she goes back to the kitchen and has half a cucumber, some leftover cold spaghetti, and an apple. Then, because she still feels dissatisfied, she finishes off some ice-cream straight from the carton, standing in front of the fridge. Then because she has blown her diet anyway she goes out and gets a pizza, and stuffs the whole thing down even though now she is not the slightest bit hungry. Obviously she would have been much better off eating the pizza in the first place.

I often hold my London weekend workshop on Finchley Road in Swiss Cottage. There is a huge selection of delis, restaurants and supermarkets, so it is really easy for the group to complete their lunchtime assignment, which is to check how hungry they are, and then go and find and eat *exactly* what they are hungry for.

It was after such a lunch-break that Andrea came rushing back into the group room. She told the group that what she had really fancied for lunch was chocolate violet creams; she had gone to an expensive chocolate shop and bought a whole pound of chocolate violet creams. Then she realized that all she liked of the chocolate was the outside. She spent the whole lunch hour nibbling the chocolate surround and throwing the centres away. Sounded fine, I thought, until I heard Andrea launch an attack on herself. 'I must be insane,' she said. 'It's crazy, who walks down the street throwing the inside of their expensive chocolate away?' I didn't think what Andrea did was crazy, and I told her so. I told her I thought that she liked to eat the outside of violet creams. Slim people have likes and dislikes too. Andrea's homework was to stock up on chocolate violet creams, to keep a permanent supply of them in the fridge, and always to throw the centre away.

In the same way that our bodies will send us a hunger signal, so too will our bodies tell us what to eat at any given moment. If you are confused about what to eat, the best thing to do is to ask. Ask you body, let your body tell you what you want.

I remember seeing a cartoon of a child going into an American ice-cream parlour, all excited about the ice-cream he is about to buy. He stands in front of the counter and greedily starts to look at the ninety-nine different flavours there are to choose from. He starts to sweat and then to shake and the last frame shows him screaming in the corner: 'I want a little bit of everything.' That is consumer terror. When we are faced with too many choices, the child in us starts to get confused. That is why we need to narrow the options down. Do you want chocolate, fruit or vanilla? Do you want chocolate chips or nuts in the ice-cream? By going through the various options and a process of elimination, it is easier to make a decision.

When You Are Hungry, How to Choose One of Ninety-Nine Different Flavours?

Food needs to be emotionally as well as physically satisfying. Each time you are hungry it will be for a particular kind of food. There is nothing more satisfying than eating *exactly* what you are hungry for. If you want something sweet, however much savoury food you eat you still won't feel satisfied. If you fancy something crunchy like toast, you won't enjoy a pot of yoghurt.

After years of dieting, we have become so out of touch with what we really like to eat, what our bodies really want, that many of us haven't got a clue what we really fancy.

To help you, here are some questions to ask yourself:

Do I want:

Hot food or cold?

Solid or liquid?

Sweet or savoury?

Crunchy or creamy?

Light or bulky?

If you trust your body it will guide you as to what and how much to eat. You have to tune inwards and listen to that inner voice. One day it will guide you to spinach and potato and the next day it may guide you to chocolate. Sometimes it will be easy to identify exactly what you want to eat, because a certain type of food will call you.

There will be times when you are not sure what you want. In such a situation, try having a conversation with yourself. Imagine that you are speaking to the 'hungry self' inside you. It may feel really awkward at first, but later it becomes much easier.

Hungry Self: I am hungry.
Me: What are you hungry for?
Hungry Self: Don't know.
Me: Something sweet or savoury?
Hungry Self: Savoury.
Me: Hot or cold?
Hungry Self: Hot.
Me: Liquid or solid?
Hungry Self: Mmmmmmmm . . . not sure. Solid.
Me: Baked potato with cheese?

Hungry Self: Sounds nice, but when I think of it in my stomach it feels too filling. I need less than that.
Me: How about a plate of pasta?
Hungry Self: Also too filling.
Me: I know you said something solid, but we could heat up the mushroom soup that I have in the fridge.
Hungry Self: Yes, just right.

Or this conversation:

Hungry Self: I am so, so hungry. I feel like eating something hot and crunchy and tasty.
Me: Toast is hot and crunchy.
Hungry Self: Yes, OK, but what can we put on it?
Me: Marmite perhaps, or peanut butter?
Hungry Self: No. I feel like something fresh and moist on the toast.
Me: Sounds like you want a lovely fresh sweet tomato.
Hungry Self: Perfect, Marmite first and then tomato, and at least two pieces.

As you are going through the options, try to imagine how the food will feel in your stomach. About a year ago, by force of circumstances, we were at a local restaurant which is famous for its fish supper. I was really hungry, and since the only dish available was fish and chips, that is what I ordered. Even though I ate only half of my food, I left feeling really uncomfortable. I felt as if I needed to drink Coke to somehow wash down the awful greasy feeling that was left in my throat. I now know that my body does not like fish suppers. I actually never feel good after too much fried food. A short while after our dinner at the fish restaurant we were out at a sports day, and the only thing available to eat was fish and chips. I remembered the awful after-taste and feeling of the fish supper, and I went across the street, where to my delight I found a sandwich shop and feasted on a brie and black grapes baguette.

When I first stopped dieting I ate all the foods I had never allowed myself previously. Whenever I was hungry I wanted pies, pastries and puddings. Then, gradually, it changed – when I knew, truly knew that I was allowed everything, I began to listen to my body more. These days, I find myself mostly choosing foods which leave me feeling good after I have eaten them.

Lillian and Leonard Pearson, authors of *The Psychologist's Eat Anything Diet*, are often quoted because they coined the words 'hummers' and 'beckoners' to describe eating different kinds of foods. Hummers are foods that we are hungry for before we see them, hear about them or smell them. We get a clear image of them in our mind and we know exactly what texture, taste and consistency they are. The sticky toffee pudding was humming to me. Nothing else would do. After I had eaten it I didn't think about or want food for the rest of the day. That is a humming food. My body had asked for it without being prompted, so it was totally satisfying to eat it.

Beckoners, on the other hand, are foods which we respond to because we see, smell or taste them. You walk into your kitchen and see a half-eaten cake and suddenly you want a slice. The half round of toast that your daughter has not eaten suddenly changes into the words 'Eat me'. You order a cup of tea in a restaurant, the waitress carries a plate of gâteau past you, and you suddenly get hungry for it. Before you saw it, you had not thought about eating, or about the cake. You were triggered to want it because you saw it, it was available, it beckoned to you. If you eat a 'beckoning' food when you are not hungry to begin with, then you will not know when to stop, and will not feel satisfied by it. Food advertisers and manufacturers know about this: they put food beckoners everywhere, on our TV screens, on billboards, at supermarket checkout counters. My aim is to eat only humming food, food that I decide I want because I am hungry for it. All other food can go and beckon somewhere else and someone else. Not me any more, thank you.

Eating what you feel like at that moment really means that. We need to love ourselves enough to take the time and trouble to eat exactly what we want. If you are hungry for apple crumble, then that is what to eat. Eating not only has to satisfy our physical hunger, it also has to be emotionally satisfying. Eating a salad when I am hungry for thick vegetable soup will take away my physical hunger but leave me needy. Don't be afraid to experiment, even if it goes against everything you have been brought up with. If you only love bread without the crusts, then leave the crusts. If you are hungry for apricot-flavoured fromage frais, don't settle for the strawberry-flavoured kind. If you dislike the nuts in the muesli, pick them out. Have exactly what you are hungry for.

The obvious question that arises is: what if I want something that is not available? After eating this way for years, I now know which foods I regularly get hungry for. I always make sure that there is a good supply of my favourite staple foods: wholemeal bread, pasta, bagels, rice, pears, bananas, fresh orange juice, tomatoes, muesli, porridge, oatcakes, McVities Boasters, peanut butter, honey and peppermint tea. If you are hungry, and you cannot get what you want, then have the closest possible alternative, to appease your hunger. Make yourself a promise that you will definitely keep – to get yourself the particular food you want at a later stage if possible.

It was during the same lunch hour when Andrea was throwing away her violet creams that I happened to overhear the conversation at the table next to mine. A slim-looking man joined two women, and he apologized for being late. The reason he gave was that he had been walking up and down looking for a special brand of Greek yoghurt. The place he usually got it from had run out, and breakfast was not breakfast without lashings of this Greek yoghurt. When he had finished his lunch he announced that he was off to another shop to see if they had the Greek yoghurt. Mmmm, yes: take time and trouble to find the foods that you love. We always made an effort to go out of our way to find the particular diet food our current diet sheet called for. We can now use that same energy to find the food we are really hungry for.

When you begin to follow this method of eating, you may need to experiment to find out what your favourite foods are.

Years following other people's diets may have made you uncertain about what you really like.

Sandra was going through a phase of being hungry for fresh hot bagels and smoked salmon. During the week she could easily get to a shop to indulge this need, but on weekends it meant making an hour-long car journey. One Saturday morning she woke hungry for a bagel, but since her husband was working in the garden and she had to take her children to soccer practice which was in the opposite direction to the bagel shop, she decided to have toast instead. Sandra made her toast and ate it and then she ate an apple, and then she ate chocolate biscuits. 'I just could not stop eating,' she said, 'until I realized that I was feeling angry and deprived. I wanted a bagel and feeding myself toast was just not enough. After soccer practice we drove to the bakery and I bought lots of bagels, two for lunch and twelve for the freezer. I ended up eating only half a bagel because I was so full of chocolate biscuits, but the half was enough. Next time I am hungry for a bagel I will go and get one.'

In Restaurants

Many people have said to me that they go into a restaurant, look at the menu, and go into a flat panic because they cannot decide what to eat. This is caused by years of living with diet mentality. The confusion is all in your own head, about calories and allowed foods and disallowed foods and heaven forbid you might put on weight. We can easily stop all that mental torture when we let our bodies decide.

Restaurants are ideal places to experiment with having exactly what you want. Before you look at the menu, ask your body what you are hungry for and then choose the nearest alternative possible. Treat the restaurant menu as a buffet table, and take as much as you are hungry for. Do not be afraid to ask for half portions, or to order only a sweet. Ask for exactly what you want, a half portion of this plus a spoon of that, please. If the food is not good, send it back. You are the customer and you are paying, you are entitled to get what you really want.

There are hundreds of restaurants in Glasgow and I have tried many of them. I only find myself going back to a restaurant if they will oblige the way that I eat. I now know that if I eat a starter, a main course and a dessert I will feel uncomfortably full, so I order what suits my appetite at that moment. Philip and I often share a course or order three starters between the two of us. Often I go to a restaurant for a specific item that I cannot buy or make myself. The scones at Café Gandolfi are in my opinion the best in town. They are hot and crunchy on the outside and soft and light on the inside. I eat them without butter and jam because they are perfect. When I am hungry for a Gandolfi scone then I make a point of going there, nothing else will do.

Variety is the Spice of Life

On a hot summer's day my body will ask for cold food and lots of liquids. On a winter's day my body wants hot steamy foods. Sometimes I am hungry for food that is bulky and at other times I want only light food. Instinctively my body really wants to be healthy, so it will often guide me to healthy food. But sometimes (especially when I am premenstrual) my body asks for sugary and buttery foods. At the beginning, I would panic as the old diet mentality reared its ugly head again. I had to learn to really listen to my body. That also meant not being scared to eat high-calorie foods when my body asked for them.

When you have trained yourself to get back in touch with your body, you will find that what you want to eat may change not only through the seasons of weather, but also through seasons in your feelings. I was spending some time with a naturally slim friend who has two young children. Over the preceding months her husband had become addicted to cocaine. We went for a walk and she cried because she felt as if she was taking care of three children. She was so needy, and all she was doing was looking after everybody else. We talked things through and then decided to go for a drink. She looked at the menu and said that she was ordering a double thick milkshake as she needed something filling and comforting. Naturally slim people do sometimes eat for reasons other than hunger – the difference between them and compulsive eaters is that they are aware that they are doing it, and it doesn't trigger a binge.

When I am tired or sad, the foods I get hungry for are different from those foods I eat when I am happy and energetic. I too sometimes eat in response to my emotions. There have been a lot of changes in my life recently. A lot of endings which have left me feeling cold inside; and a lot of new beginnings which make me feel frightened. As these feelings intensified, the food I got hungry for changed. I wanted foods that were filling and comforting – fluffy baked potatoes, creamy mushroom soup and hot milky drinks.

Food choices change with my feelings. This is different from eating compulsively to stuff down my feelings, this is eating when I am hungry in accordance with the way I am feeling and what my body needs.

Bringing Forbidden Foods Back into Your Life

Eating what you want means eating exactly what you want – whether it is salad and pasta, or doughnuts and chocolate. Whenever I say that to a group for the first time, all hell breaks loose. Somebody always says that if she allowed herself to eat what she wanted, all she would eat is piles of junk food, because that is all she thinks and dreams about. And, yes, at the beginning, once you have decided to trust yourself enough to eat the exact thing that you are hungry for, that is exactly what may happen. The longer we go without something the more bewitching it becomes. If you have spent years telling yourself that cake and cream, butter and bacon are definitely not allowed, then these foods will be highly charged in your imagination.

When I was eighteen I met Mark. He was ten years older

than me, had graduated from university and was living with his girlfriend. I was absolutely thunderstruck. He was the knight in shining armour who would carry me off into the sunset. We would get married and I would be a beautiful, and of course thin, bride. For three years I dreamed about being with him, fantasized about how magnificent he was, how he knew everything and how wonderful we would be together. No other man would do, nobody could compare to Mark. If only he was available, if only the girlfriend would disappear.

I was ecstatic to hear one day that his relationship had ended. I finally plucked up courage to ask him out on a date, and spent the whole day getting ready for it. But what a shock – all that I found across the dinner table was a very boring man! He spoke about only one thing, himself. There was an even bigger shock in store for me when he kissed me, because there was no earthquake, not even one little bolt of lightning. The Mark that I had created in my imagination did not exist: what made him so exciting was that he was unobtainable. When he phoned for another date, I said no.

We always want what we have been told we cannot have. Cream cakes, nutty chocolate, crisps, fresh Danish pastry. Any food on the No No diet list is likely to conjure up images of ecstasy. The foods that we are not allowed become our master. Because we cannot have them we want them, and the more we don't have them the more we want them, lots and lots of them. Perhaps chocolate will never be as boring as Mark was, but now that I have eaten chocolate, with full permission, hundreds of times, it is just chocolate. And apples are just apples too.

Our aim in this exercise is to feel safe and free around food in any context. If you are faced with the choice between chocolate cake, a cheese sandwich and celery sticks, I want you to be able to let your body hunger direct your food choice. Thoughts of calories should have nothing to do with your choice. If you listen, I mean really listen to your body, the choice will be an easy one.

It is important that you bring back into your life all the

foods that have been previously forbidden. If pudding has been banned from your life for years, you may initially always be hungry for pudding. Wanting lots and lots of pudding is only a phase, and it will pass. I can assure you that eventually your body will just have had enough of the butter and sugar and rich pudding ingredients.

Often, during this initial phase of reintroducing all foods into their lives, Weigh Ahead participants get very worried about their health and nutrition. But I tell them, yes, it is unhealthy to live on chips and chocolate for ever, but it is also really unhealthy to keep up the diet–binge syndrome with weight fluctuations. You have been dieting and bingeing for years. I know that after a few weeks of chips and chocolate your body is going to want salad. I believe that the body's natural trend is towards health. If you take the risk and allow the time it takes for fries and fresh cream to lose their naughty, forbidden appeal, they will eventually become as neutral as apples and pears. More often than not you will end up wanting and enjoying pears most of the time, and only the occasional dollop of cream.

The forbidden foods that have cropped up most often for my Weigh Ahead participants have been bread, crisps, and, most of all, chocolate. I remember one woman in particular who introduced herself to the group by talking about her struggle with chocolate. Betty would not allow herself any for weeks, and then she would binge on bars and boxes of it.

Her homework was to go and buy all her favourite chocolates – much more than she could possibly eat in a week. Every time she was hungry for chocolate, she was to eat some. After a few weeks, she reported back to the group: 'The first day all I ate was chocolate for breakfast, tea, lunch and dinner. I kept on opening the cupboard and looking at all the chocolate. It was amazing, like a dream. All this chocolate, and Cherie says I am allowed as much as I am hungry for.

'The second day my husband thought I was going crazy. I set the table with our best dinner service and cooked a delicious meal for the family. Then I arranged a selection of

Ferrero Rocher chocolates on my plate, and that's all I had for supper.

'But after three days of chocolate I suddenly began to notice something. Chocolate is very, very sweet. I began to feel like real food, so I made myself a baked potato and ate half of it; then I had a mini Snickers bar. By the fifth day, I was only opening my chocolate cupboard once a day. I still have a cupboard full of chocolate, I eat a bit every now and again. I cannot believe it: me with a cupboard full of chocolate, and I hardly even think about it. Now, when I feel like chocolate, I know where to find it, and I have some.'

When you approach a box of chocolates with the thought, 'I am not allowed these, I shouldn't have these,' you will want the whole box. If you approach the chocolate with the thought that you are allowed as much as you are hungry for, then you are in control, and you have choice. You then only need eat as much as you are hungry for.

If initially ice-cream is all you are hungry for, then eat ice-cream until your body decides it has had enough. Once the deprivation, the famine you have imposed on your body is over, once all foods are neutral, it will signal for salad or fruit. But first you have to allow the time it takes for the foods that you were not allowed while dieting to lose their forbidden appeal.

When you are eating more spontaneously, there may come a time when you wish to address the issue of nutrition. But in the early stages of stopping compulsive overeating I suggest that for however long it takes you allow yourself whatever you are hungry for. Try and differentiate between wanting food because you were never allowed it, or wanting food because you are hungry for it now, at this minute.

If the thought of bringing all foods back into your life is scary, then do it slowly, and gradually. Make a list of all the foods that you never allow yourself, and rank them from your most favourite to your least favourite. When you are hungry, reintroduce all the forbidden foods one by one, say once a week, beginning at the top of your list. Reassure yourself with the fact that one bar of chocolate, or a slice of cake, or a plate of pudding, won't make you put on weight overnight. Rather think of how relaxing it will be to live without the rigidity and control you have always placed yourself under.

During a workshop we always have a meal together. Everybody brings their favourite main course or pudding to share. After the meal everybody takes back what is left of the dishes they brought. One night, while everybody was getting ready to leave, Joan came up to me with half a chocolate cheesecake. 'I want to leave this here,' she said. 'If I take this home I will eat the whole thing tonight. There is no way I can leave a chocolate cheesecake in my fridge and not finish it.'

The whole group knew who Joan was, even before she introduced herself at the start of the workshop. She had been named businesswoman of the year in 1993 in the city where she lived. The retail organization she had begun ten years ago now employed over 300 people, and she was currently planning two new outlets in another city. She also ran a large home for her husband and three children, and regularly worked for a charity. I stood there thinking that the power we let food have over us is amazing. Here was a successful, outstanding woman who trusted herself enough to deal with employees, tax officials, bank managers and a business which turned over millions of pounds. She trusted herself enough to do all that, trusted herself to be an excellent mother and wife, but she did not trust herself enough to have chocolate cheesecake in her fridge.

Food has no power except the power that we give it. If we trust ourselves, I mean really trust ourselves, then we can begin to take back the power we have always given to food. Trusting yourself means taking the chocolate cheesecake home and knowing that you can eat a piece when you are hungry for some. Being scared of having the chocolate cheesecake at home means you don't trust yourself. People who are told they cannot be trusted become defiant, and it is this defiance which sends us chomping through whatever is left of what we have been told we cannot have. Not trusting yourself to have food in your home means you are committing yourself to a life of deprivation and bingeing. If you cannot learn to trust yourself, then if by chance the 'forbidden' item is in your home it will develop a voice and call to you: 'I am so close, come eat me. I am here waiting, eat me.' So you binge on it, finish it, feel sick and hate yourself.

But if you get used to living with cheesecake in the fridge, and chocolates and biscuits in the cupboard, then you need only eat these when you are hungry for them. Allow yourself to have these 'naughty' foods around. As much as you can afford. Eventually you will get so used to having them in the house you will only think of them when you are hungry for them.

P.S. I convinced Joan that she should always leave a chocolate cheesecake in her fridge, a large one. When it was almost finished, she was to bake another one. The last time I spoke to her Joan said she was tired of the taste of chocolate cheesecake and the last one she made went mouldy before she remembered it.

P.P.S. *Of course it goes without saying that if you are diabetic, suffer from high cholesterol or have any other medical condition that is affected by what you eat, you must follow your doctor's advice, and avoid eating foods that would be dangerous to your health.*

Some common questions:
My wife has just lost a stone on a diet, she weighs and measures her food and says I am crazy, that I will never lose weight without dieting. She does not want me to stock up with chocolate because she gets tempted, in fact the whole thing is causing a lot of tension.
Unfortunately this problem can often arise. You tell your friends and family that you are giving up dieting and that you are going to eat when you are hungry and they look at you as if you are crazy. You are three stone overweight and eating sticky toffee pudding; they think that overweight

people should live on carrots. Explain this programme and hope for some understanding. If your friends or partner still want to continue dieting, that is their choice. Your choice is not to diet, and just as you will allow them their choice, they must allow you yours.

With regard to having different food in the house, talk to each other about a solution in which everybody's needs can be met. If your spouse does not want chocolate in the house, then agree that you will keep chocolate in a place that she does not know about. Try and reach a solution that suits both of you.

What do I do with my children, they would eat sweets all the time if I let them?

If your children are old enough you can talk to them about hunger and eating healthily, and let them participate in shopping and choosing what they want to eat. Allow them to get to know their own body signals, and to eat their favourite foods. Children can be very specific: 'I want one and a half sausages, a bread roll and three green beans, please.' Children's appetites vary from day to day.

Unfortunately children have an appetite for junk food, so we have to set limits for them, and they also need freedom to experiment within those limits. Explain why it is not good to eat three chocolates instead of dinner, but also allow them to have some chocolate if they are hungry for it, after dinner. Make the study of nutrition interesting and not a chore. Be careful not to make sweets and chocolates into 'deprived, forbidden foods'; let sweets be as neutral as fruit is. Have fun with fruit and veg – cut faces, and make shapes. Put nuts and raisins in their packed lunch one day; the next day put in crisps, the next fruit and the next chocolate.

The best thing you can do for your children is to work on your own eating problem. I know that the last thing in the world you want is for your child to become a compulsive eater. But our children learn their eating behaviour from us. They pick up our habits, our prejudices. Unfortunately food often becomes the battleground on which the battle for independence and separation is fought. Mothers especially can become too involved in whether junior eats up all his food. And he knows this, so there is much to be gained by him for not eating. If your child is full of energy, playing, going to school, then probably he is fine, even if he is living on toast and cheese alone, or nothing but oranges and chocolate. Defocus your attention and trust him to eat when he is hungry, just as you are trusting yourself to. When the weekly diet of even the faddiest child is diagnosed, it usually shows that in spite of what you think it is reasonably balanced.

If children are provided with the safe, supportive and consistent loving which they all deserve, they are free to grow up without the vacuum that we as compulsive eaters always try to fill with food.

3. Seeing, Smelling, Tasting and Enjoying

Hiding from Ourselves

I was watching an overweight young girl eating on the train. She sat down with a Kit Kat, a magazine and a bag of crisps. She unwrapped the chocolate, opened the bag of crisps and began reading the magazine. She ate as she was reading, and only seemed to become aware that she had finished the food when she tapped down on the empty bag and wrappers. When the food trolley came down the aisle she bought a packet of biscuits and ate them in exactly the same absent-minded way. She did not seem to taste or enjoy the food; she might as well have been sleeping while someone else spooned the food into her mouth.

Sitting opposite the young girl on the train was a slim man who had also bought a Kit Kat. He put down his paper, unwrapped the chocolate and broke each finger in half. He picked up a piece and ate it slowly. In between bites he stopped eating and read his newspaper. When he was eating the chocolate he stopped reading. He made his Kit Kat last longer than the crisps, the Kit Kat and the packet of biscuits of the girl I was watching. It isn't hard to guess which of them was naturally slim.

A lot of the people who come to my workshops say that they really love eating. But when I ask them about their eating habits, about when and how they eat, I hear the following – I eat food out of the pot while I am cooking, I stand and eat food straight out of the fridge, I sneak into the kitchen for a biscuit, I eat in the car, in the street, I can't watch TV or read the paper without eating something, I finish the children's leftover fish fingers, I straighten the way a cake has been cut. I recognize these habits: that is the way I fed myself for ages. That is not proper eating with enjoyment, that is hiding from yourself while you are eating. And I ask them, as I once asked myself, why are you hiding from yourself?

When we are eating we are providing nourishment for ourselves, we are giving ourselves the energy we require to live. Think of the trouble we go to for dinner party guests, with the table beautifully laid and all the food attractively prepared in advance. We sit down with our guests, the candles are lit, and the food is savoured and complimented. This is the way we must also feed ourselves.

Many of the people I work with feel guilty after every morsel they put into their mouth. Eating is always accompanied by judgemental thoughts: either I am allowed this, or I am not allowed this. We need to expand the permission we have given ourselves to eat forbidden foods even further, and give ourselves full permission to eat all food. We are allowed to eat. If we do not eat we will die. We need to eat everyday, for the rest of our lives.

If you wake up every morning with the idea that the only food that is permissible is your low-calorie allowance, it immediately sets up the tug-of-war which causes us to overeat. When we do eat we feel guilty. We eat without real enjoyment, we sneak the food, not only from others but also from ourselves.

Sneak eating is a good way of pretending that we are not eating. If I sneak into the kitchen for a biscuit, then another and another, I can eat ten biscuits without realizing it. If I sat down with a plate and two biscuits, and I savoured them, enjoyed them, I wouldn't feel the need to keep going back for more. Sneak eating means depriving yourself of the enjoyment of eating, so you won't feel satisfied — and you will go on eating.

If what we say is true, that is, that we love eating, then why do we eat the way we do? How can I love something if I don't give it time and attention? If I gobble a piece of toast while I am rushing off to work, I will not taste or enjoy that piece of toast. If I eat a chocolate in the car while I am concentrating on changing lanes I won't even notice I'm eating something. If I wasn't driving, I could unwrap the chocolate slowly, look at it, nibble at the edge, lick the filling in the centre, savour, taste and enjoy the chocolate; I would be aware that I was eating it, would love eating it. If I put the piece of toast on a plate, sit down, cut it into pieces and eat slowly, I will taste it, be aware that I have eaten it. And if I am aware, really aware, that I have eaten something, if I have tasted it, crunched it, and enjoyed every mouthful, I will feel aware of my body, that I feel satisfied. I will feel nourished. And if I feel nourished, I am less likely to want more of what I am eating.

Practising Nourishing Eating

Here are some guidelines I use myself and which I recommend to participants in my workshops. They are guidelines which will help to focus your attention on your eating and help you to get in touch with your hunger — so that you can feed yourself in a nourishing way.

- *Never eat anything standing up*. Whatever it is that you are eating, SIT DOWN. Even binge food, or the remains of your child's noodle doodles. Sit down.

- *Always, always eat off a plate.* Biscuit, fruit, crisps, or peanuts
  – whatever it is, put it on a plate and eat it with attention,
  it will be much more enjoyable that way, and you are much
  less likely to eat unconsciously. Both this suggestion and the
  previous one will help you cut down on unconscious eating.
  You know the bits of food that somehow you never ate but
  which magically appear on your hips and stomach. If you put
  all the food you are about to eat on a plate and sit down, you
  are immediately changing your habit of unconscious eating.
- *Be your own guest.* Whenever you can, set the table, use
  crockery and cutlery that you enjoy looking at. Sit in a
  comfortable chair, play nice soft music in the background
  perhaps, and begin to eat. That is what someone who really
  loves eating will do.
- *Don't distract yourself.* Don't eat in the car, on public
  transport, in the street. Don't read or watch TV while you
  are eating. Eating can be one of those times when you stop
  rushing, and doing. A time to enjoy being with yourself. A
  time to focus all your attention on the food you are eating.
  If, as you say, eating is so important, then why do you have
  to escape from eating by reading and watching TV at the same
  time? Why do you gobble your sandwich in the car while you
  are concentrating on the traffic? It always astonishes me how
  difficult Weigh Ahead participants find this: for years, they
  have been hoovering up food while focusing their attention
  elsewhere. So many times I have heard: 'I've got to have the
  TV on while I'm eating,' or 'I *can't* eat without reading the
  paper.' The point is, when you are eating, then eat and give
  it your full attention, and when you are reading, read and
  enjoy that.
- *Give yourself permission to enjoy what you are about to eat.*
  I really mean that, permission to eat with gusto. Permission
  to delight in the food. Once you have begun eating, be aware
  of the food in your mouth. Notice the process of eating,
  chewing, and tasting. Actually say the words to yourself:
  I'M EATING, I'M CHEWING, I'M TASTING. Get sensual

about the flavours and textures. Notice the subtlety of the different flavours. Try and guess what ingredients are in the food, identify the separate herbs and spices. Crunch, chew and roll the food around with your tongue. Feel the sensation of having your mouth filled with food. Taste it, really taste it. Notice the difference in the initial and the after taste. Get sensual about the food, roll it, lick it and really enjoy it. Notice the food at your throat as you swallow. And notice the difference in your stomach as the food you have chewed and swallowed reaches it.

• *Avoid emotional conversations while eating.* If you know you have something important to discuss, try not to do it over a meal. Emotional conversations are bound to stir up pain and/or anger within yourself and this will seriously affect the way you eat. If the conversation suddenly becomes heated during a meal, put your knife and fork down. You can eat later when the food is not smothered by the feelings.

No Need to Sneak: Hiding from Others

Because of the fattist society that we live in, people who are overweight are often made to feel as if they have no right to eat in front of others. We do have the right to eat. No matter how overweight we are, we still get hungry, and when we are hungry we need to eat. We have the right to eat with enjoyment in front of other people.

Being naturally slim is a state of mind; within this state of mind food and eating are totally neutral. Like breathing is. Food is eaten and prepared every day and whenever it is necessary. Food and eating are an accepted part of being alive.

Jack remembers school dinners because he and three of the other boys at his school who were also on a diet had to sit at a special table and eat salad. Every day without fail, lunch for them consisted of salad, fruit instead of dessert and a full helping of jeers from the others boys. Hey, fatso, blubberboat. Watch out here come the floorbreakers. All this was a lesson in how to break a little boy's heart. Jack says he found a way to make himself feel better: he would always arrive at school really early and he would sneak into the staff tearoom and take one round of sandwiches from each of the six plates of sandwiches. Those he could not eat immediately he would hide in his desk, and every time he thought of the salad table he would eat a sandwich and promise himself that when he was older he was going to eat as much as he possibly could. He would show them. Unfortunately he needed to show them so badly that he now weighs over twenty stone.

One day, before the start of a workshop, my group and I were having coffee and biscuits. I returned from another room to the table where the refreshments were, just at the moment when one of the participants was taking two chocolate biscuits. She was startled when she noticed me, and she guiltily launched into an explanation. She had just come back from work, and she had had no time for lunch, and since the group was three hours long she needed something to eat now. 'Are you hungry for a chocolate biscuit?' I asked her. 'Yes,' she replied, and I said, 'Well that's fine, then why fuss?'

Nowadays when I am hungry I eat, and I do not need to give anybody an excuse about it. I am in control. I decide. It has not always been that way though – I used to eat 'like a bird' in front of people. Then when I got home I would literally attack the refrigerator. I believed that nobody should ever see me eating, but they did, I got caught a few times and the shame of that still burns in my memory.

Arnold, my first boyfriend, had come with me to a party at my eldest sister's house. Before we left I had eaten my Weight Watchers dinner, and had taken an apple with me for later. At midnight, after we had been dancing for hours, I was starving, ravenous. I wandered over to the food table and decided that I would pretend it was breakfast and have a bread roll with egg salad, and then not eat until lunch-time the next day. Once I had tasted the roll, however, I knew one would not be enough – I had another, and another, and then nibbled at some of the other dishes. I went back to the room and found Arnold, who said to me, 'I could see into the dining-room and I have been sitting here watching you eating like a pig!' I was mortified, what a mistake!

Just as bad was the time I got caught eating pudding at another party. I was not going to have any, but then found myself unable to resist. I waited until there was nobody around the pudding table. I went over and filled my plate, then sat down and ate it as quickly as possible before anybody could see me. I looked up and to my horror not only had somebody seen me – *I had been filmed*. The photographer who was taking a video of the party had filmed the whole scene. I was even more humiliated when the film was played back to the people who had stayed late. The shame that I felt that night stayed with me for weeks after. Everybody had seen me, the fat person, committing the worst sin of all – eating.

We have all been conditioned by our fattist society into the assumption that all overweight people must be on a diet. In fact that *all* women are probably on a diet, fat or thin. It is just not acceptable for a woman to tuck into food with relish in public. Marianne, my editor, reminded me about Scarlett's Mammy, in *Gone With the Wind*, who makes Scarlett eat something before the party so that she will be able to eat daintily – like a lady – at the party. Well, since those days which Margaret Mitchell wrote about we have seen women burn their bras and throw away their girdles, but we still feel ashamed of being seen eating in public.

If you are hungry and have decided what it is you want to eat then sit down, put your food on to a plate, and eat with relish. Ooh and aaah about the food, savour it, roll it around your mouth.

Eat in front of anybody, and with the intention of being seen by everybody. You are allowed to eat. If somebody you live with gives you a hard time, talk it through with them, tell them about this programme and that you are now responsible for what and how much you eat. Tell them that it really bothers you when they comment on your eating, and they should back off, please. You are in control, and you do not, ever, need to apologize for eating. Not ever.

4. Stopping When You Are Satisfied

I hope you have been observing naturally slim people since you have been reading this book, because they are our role models. There is a way you can immediately tell if a person is naturally slim or not. If they usually leave food behind on their plate, they are probably naturally slim. Have you noticed that? Even if they love the food they are eating, they seem to be able to leave a bite or two, or even half their portion behind. Naturally slim people stop eating when they are satisfied. That means they govern the amount that they eat by listening to their bodies, and not by how much is left on their plate. Luckily for them, they do not feel compelled to overeat when they feel satisfied, they can stop eating, and think no more of it. Naturally slim people say things like, 'No more for me, thank you. It was delicious, but I'm full up. I couldn't eat another morsel.' In the past such utterances would baffle me. I often felt stuffed – but it never prevented me from continuing to eat.

Imagine the scenario – two people eating equal portions of chicken pie. One person eats three-quarters of her pie, sighs, pushes her plate away and relaxes. The other person eats half her piece of pie, then, as she starts thinking about all the calories in the pastry, all the fat in the sauce, she tenses, her hand to mouth movements become faster, and faster. She cannot stop herself and she finishes every last scrap of pie, and scrapes the plate. Then she starts to criticize herself, she calls herself a greedy guts and starts to make promises about the diet which will start tomorrow. She leaves the table feeling stuffed, uncomfortable, depressed, hating herself. She wants to eat something else to make herself feel better.

Naturally slim people simply stop eating when they are satisfied. We dieters and overeaters have to contend with the barrage of thoughts that we live with: calories, losing weight, wanting to stop and not being able to, screaming at ourselves when we feel we have overeaten, or in fact screaming at ourselves every time we eat.

If you want your weight to stabilize you need to learn to stop when you are satisfied – but that barrage of thoughts is not going to go away overnight. First you need to be aware of it. As you are eating, monitor your thoughts, and as soon as the calorie-counting and criticisms begin, mentally shout STOP. Remind yourself you are learning to be naturally slim, that you are entitled to eat until you feel satisfied.

Because my son, Alan, cannot speak properly, the signal he uses to tell us he has had enough is that he touches his head, he brings his little hand up to his forehead and that means stop feeding me please, I have had enough. Sometimes he finishes every last scrap of food on his plate and sometimes he leaves three-quarters of it behind. He knows to the exact last mouthful when he has had enough. He loves Twirls – sometimes in three bites he devours the whole chocolate, but sometimes he leaves some behind. One bite of chocolate left, but he has had enough so he leaves it. In my dieting days, I would have found it unthinkable to leave anything. He does not think about it, he feels it in his body, he knows that one more bite will be too much.

I was so proud that he had learnt the signal and yet I nearly ruined it, because there would be times when he would touch his head and I would look at the plateful of vegetables and start playing little games: just three more bites, Alan, look, here's an aeroplane, it is flying into your mouth, please, just three more bites. But I knew that he ate his vegetables when he was hungry for them. I had to remind myself not to teach him to eat when he was not hungry; he has a signal, a little voice inside him that says enough, I have had enough.

For many of us the problem started in childhood. Like Alan,

you tried to stop when you had had enough, but your parents wouldn't let you. They told you to finish eating everything on your plate, to think of the starving children in Africa or Asia; perhaps they told you that you were selfish and spoiled and that when they were children they would have been thrilled to have all this lovely food that Mummy had cooked specially for you. You learnt that being good meant ignoring that little voice that told you you were full up, that you had had enough. And then you lost the sound of that little voice altogether.

Try to listen to that quiet little voice. A voice which will say, enough now, thank you. It does not matter if there is half a roast potato or three-quarters of a piece of pie left. The voice will say enough, I have had enough. To hear that voice you need to listen very carefully for it. Perhaps it will be a whisper, or a deep breath. But you can only hear it if you listen for it. You can only hear it if you choose to.

During a meal when you get the 'satisfied' signal you have a choice: you can choose to listen, and to stop eating, or you can choose to ignore it, and continue to eat. For a naturally slim person that choice is easy, for a compulsive eater it is not. Stopping when you are satisfied means saying no to the comfort, and the calming effect, that food provides. So you have to learn to get that comfort and calm elsewhere.

Here are some suggestions to help you learn when you have had enough, and how to stop eating when you do reach that point:

1. *Pay attention to what you are eating.* If I am watching TV, or driving, or reading, or having an argument, I am going to miss the signal to stop when I am satisfied. I hear such complaints when I advise people not to eat and read or eat and watch TV: 'Lunch is not lunch without the *Independent*,' or 'I cannot eat alone without watching the news.'

   You need to concentrate on what you are eating so that you can stop when you are satisfied, and also be aware that you have eaten.

2. *Eat slowly.* Very slowly. I know this is difficult to do after a lifetime of eating too quickly. It takes twenty minutes after we have eaten something for the food to be absorbed into our stomachs. What happens is that as you chew, the enzymes in your saliva start working to break down the food. When the food reaches your stomach more enzymes are released and these, together with your stomach acid, begin their work of digesting the food. Only after this do the nutrients in the food start to be absorbed into your bloodstream. As the remaining food passes from your stomach into your small intestines, more of it is absorbed. The blood from your stomach and small intestine travels in your bloodstream to your brain. In your brain there is a special centre, called the satiety centre, and it is this satiety centre, together with the stretch receptors which are located in your stomach wall, which sends you the signal that you have eaten enough. I can eat three sandwiches and two chocolate bars in five minutes flat. Twenty minutes later, I will feel uncomfortable and so full. If I eat one sandwich and one chocolate bar slowly, chewing, tasting and stopping between bites, I will allow myself to know when I am satisfied.

3. *Be aware of any change in the taste of the food you are eating.* If you concentrate on the taste you will notice at a particular moment a change in the taste of what you are eating. This is another message from your body, a message you will never have heard in the years of dieting and overeating. At this point ask yourself, 'Am I still hungry,' and if you are, perhaps it is time for a different food, because the message from you body means, 'I have had enough of that particular food.'

4. *Be aware of the feeling within as the food reaches your stomach.* Each few mouthfuls will change your hunger sensation and you need to be aware of this. You need to tune inward to really listen for that moment when it is time to stop. The best way to check on your hunger level is to stop eating for a moment. Put down your knife and

fork, and when you have swallowed the food that is in your mouth, take a deep breath in, and breathe out slowly. On the out breath ask yourself how hungry you are. Compare it to how hungry you were at the start of the meal. This requires a lot of concentration initially, but quickly becomes easier, and you will find yourself doing it almost automatically.

5. *Before eating, decide approximately how much you think you need to satisfy your hunger.* Then insert some imaginary commas and a full stop in your meal. For example, I am hungry for a sandwich and a piece of fruit. My commas will be at the end of each half sandwich, and the full stop after the banana. At all my punctuation marks I will stop and check on my hunger level. Stop when you are satisfied. Reassure yourself that it is all right to stop eating because you will eat again as soon as you are hungry.

6. *If you are not sure if you are satisfied or not,* allow yourself two more bites, and then check again; or you can get up from the table and walk around, and then see if you are still hungry.

7. *If you are not hungry any more,* and you are staying at the table, get rid of any food left in front of you, don't leave it to beckon you. Wrap it up or throw it away.

8. *Plan what you are going to do after you stop eating.* Avoid hanging around at the table and the temptation to go on eating. Arrange some activity so that you have some reason to leave the table, even if it is just to brush your teeth or do the washing up.

9. *Reassure yourself that you are never ever going to force yourself to go hungry again.* Often we do not want to stop eating because of all our years of deprivation. Promise yourself that if you are hungry again in an hour, you can eat something then. Remember it takes twenty minutes for the message that food has been eaten to reach your brain. When the food has had more time to be absorbed, you will probably not feel hungry any more, but if you *are* hungry in an hour *be sure* to honour your promise and eat something. After all, it is important that you learn to trust yourself again.

This is what Alison wrote to me:

'I woke up on Thursday morning and I felt really anxious. I was not dieting, but because I now knew what body hunger was, I had decided to wait until I was hungry before I could eat. Part of me felt this was just like dieting. I went into the kitchen and looked at my cupboards full of sweets, chocolates, bread and biscuits and constantly reminded myself that I could eat as soon as I was hungry. I made myself a cup of tea but I just could not settle, so I decided to go for a walk. The air was crisp and clean, a new day in which to start my new life. I walked down Gibson Street and before I knew it I was standing in front of the shop window at my local bakery. Since I started on your programme the food in there has looked very different because I am allowed to have it. Even so I played a game with myself and I wondered if I should eat a few doughnuts, and start waiting for my hunger tomorrow. I laughed out loud as I heard myself going down that well worn track, a road that I have been on so many times before, always without any success. I turned around and went back home.

At five past eleven, at last, I felt it, yes, a real rumbling just behind my belly button, I waited another ten minutes to be sure and there it was, real hunger like welcoming a friend, a long-lost friend. I ate a piece of toast with butter and honey and it tasted marvellous. I got hungry again at two and then at seven, I skated through the day. I ate more than when I was dieting and much less than when I was not dieting. I was scared and I enjoyed it. This is a new day and tomorrow will be a new day. Tomorrow I will get hungry and I will eat only when I am hungry. I never need to go hungry again, I celebrate my hunger and I look forward to getting hungry every new day.

I love living this way. Thank you.

Love, Alison.

The Meal

I have spent a lot of time describing to you how to go about eating as naturally slim people do. I know that 'practice makes perfect', so in my workshop I always have a group meal so that we can practise eating what we want and stopping when we are satisfied.

My first experience of a group meal was the dinner I attended which was part of Maureen Kark's Weight Winners programme in South Africa.

We each brought our favourite dish to the meal. Before we began the meal, Maureen told us to close our eyes and place our hands on the place where we experienced hunger. I peeped through half-closed eyes and noticed that some people had their hands on their throats, some on their heads, and most on various places on their abdomens. Then we concentrated on giving our hunger a number. We were instructed to go over to the food and help ourselves to everything that looked nice. This meant filling three plates, for all three courses at the same time, and taking them back to our seats.

Even though we were dying to start, we waited for the next instruction: we began to examine all the items of food in front of us: we were asked to notice the colour, the shape, the consistency. Finally, we were told to take one bite of what looked like our favourite food. We were asked to really taste, chew, and savour the food before we swallowed it. When I looked at all the different foods in front of me, the one that sprang to life for me was the garlic bread. It was white with a golden crust and in the centre I could see lashings of garlic and parsley over the golden melted butter. I took a bite and enjoyed the pungent taste of garlic as it hit my taste buds. The next exercise was to smell every item of food on our plates and then take another single bite. It was hilarious watching everybody pick up their plates and smell the food, but it was also enlightening to notice how different everything smelled. This time the aroma of the tomato called me – it smelled so fresh

I just knew I wanted some. That was the first time in my life I really tasted a tomato, the fresh wet seedy taste was fantastic. After I had swallowed it my mouth felt so fresh and clean.

The next instruction from Maureen was that we should take one small bite of every different kind of food on our starter, main course and pudding plates. After each bite we had to put down our knife, fork and spoon, and chew and eat really slowly, savouring and tasting each and every bite. There was silence as we tasted our way through all the various dishes that had been brought to the meal. I tasted my foods in the order that I would have normally eaten them – starter, then main course and salad, and finally dessert.

We were then told to decide what our favourite food of that moment was. Because that was what we were going to eat next. It did not matter if our favourite food was a dessert, we were told to eat what we were most hungry for right now. It was easy for me to decide, because I had tasted the rice pudding. It was creamy and had loads of sultanas and cinnamon. My stomach told me that the rice pudding was exactly what I wanted. I ate about five spoonfuls of it. Slowly. I put my spoon down between bites. The person sitting next to me had chosen to eat lasagne.

Several times through the meal Maureen stopped us and we repeated the initial hunger exercise. We closed our eyes, put our hands on the place where we experienced hunger, and gave our hunger a new number. I began the meal with my hunger at level 2. Then, after the initial tasting and spoons of rice pudding, my hunger level had dropped to number 4. I was so surprised, and secretly disappointed. I had imagined it would take a lot more food than it did to get to number 4 and I still wanted to eat some of the other dishes. I began to eat some chicken curry, and again was so delighted at the way I could celebrate the taste of what I was eating. When I was eating compulsively I never used to taste my food; I ate it as if I was scared of it and had to get rid of it as quickly as possible.

By the next time we did the hunger exercise, I knew I was satisfied, and I felt amazed as I looked at how much food was still left on my three plates. That for me was the biggest breakthrough that night, how little food I needed to satisfy my hunger, and how incredibly delicious it tasted when I ate it slowly. Many people did not find it as easy as I did to stop eating when they were satisfied. They felt deprived because they had not seen so much lovely food for ages. Others were very upset at the amount of food that would be wasted. These were all members of the clean plate club – taught to finish every last scrap of food because of all the starving children in the world, their mothers made them do it when they were children and now they make themselves do it. Somebody complained about the sheer waste of food and Maureen replied: 'Well, what would you rather do, throw away the food in the bin or throw away the food down your throat? That is what we do when we eat when we are not hungry, we waste the food. Eating up the leftovers of the kids' fish fingers is like turning ourselves into a dustbin. We would waste less if we started a compost heap, saved it for the dog, served smaller portions. Why treat yourself as a dustbin?'

Before we lined up in front of the two black bin bags and threw the food that was left on our plates away, we did two exercises that Bob Schwartz describes in *Diets Don't Work*. The first exercise was to play with our food, like children, to mess it around with our fingers, even throw it. It was a real insight to do this: first, the food that looked so wonderful did not do so when it was all mushed and squirted around, and second, it was great fun. Also the food lost its mystique: it was only food. But some people found this extremely difficult to do, and became upset. When they discussed their reaction later, it came out that they had been taught as children that food was to be taken seriously and never played with, never wasted.

Next, we were all told to make a fist and hold it up in the air. I looked at the fist I had made and I could guess what was coming next: the size of my fist is the size of my stomach when it is empty. Of course it can stretch to become much larger than that, but it really does not take that many bites to fill it.

I loved this meal and later integrated it into my own programme. The Weigh Ahead group meal is always an important event. Everybody brings a dish of their favourite food, and the table usually groans with a wide variety: from chicken salad and broccoli bake, to brie, chocolate mousse and creamy trifle. We all bring our best crockery and cutlery and we set the table with flowers and candlelight. There is a choice of wine and soft drinks, and it turns into a sort of dinner party.

I am always touched by the atmosphere at the meal. There is joy and excitement about; these people tend to adore food, yet fear eating. People know that they are about to embark on a new and different journey. Nothing on the table is disallowed, we have total freedom to eat exactly what and how much we want . . .

Dear Cherie
I have just arrived back home after participating in the meal at your workshop. I am so excited, I will not even attempt to sleep. I have decided to write to you instead.

When the session began, and everybody described what they had brought to eat, I was terrified. I could smell the garlic bread, I had seen the cream and chocolate. I was so hungry, I just did not know how I would manage to stop when I was satisfied, not with all that delicious food in abundance.

When you told us to walk around and look at the different foods it was an amazing experience. I have never looked at the colour, and texture and shape of food before. The tomato seemed redder than red, the chicken looked drab and brown. From the minute I saw the chocolate biscuit pudding, it began to dance. It looked rich and dark and I knew I was going to have some for dessert.

Imagine my surprise when you told us to begin our meal with the foods which looked the most inviting. I agree that it is only tradition which dictates that we should eat our meat, three veg and salad before pudding. I was hungry for the chocolate biscuit pudding at the start of the meal; if I had ploughed through the starter, and main course, I would have been too full to enjoy my pudding.

We began the meal by eating our favourite food, slowly. Each mouthful was to be savoured, indulged in and really tasted. I really did enjoy every rich, chocolatey mouthful. I got sensual about the food which I ate tonight. I rolled it around my mouth, I enjoyed biting down on to it, I imagined what ingredients were in it. The pudding tasted heavenly.

It was difficult for me to put my spoon down between bites. I kept on forgetting. I know I will really need to concentrate on not shovelling my food in any more. I have been eating that way for years.

I want to tell you that I stuck to the contract that we all made at the start of the meal, and I did not overeat tonight. It really helped when we stopped several times throughout the meal and did a quick check on our hunger level.

After the pudding I had gone on to eating cheese and biscuits. (Yes, I am making up for three years of eating fat-free, and getting fatter.) There were four biscuits with a variety of cheeses on my plate, and I was munching my way through them, when you stopped us again and asked how hungry we were. I was shocked, because I knew my hunger was gone, and I had eaten enough. I looked at the food still on my plate. I felt sad, and I wished I could carry on eating.

I noticed what was happening to the people around me. For some people the fact that they had the choice to stop, or not stop, eating was enough, and they pushed their plates away easily, when they were satisfied.

For others like me who keep their cupboards at home devoid of delicious food, it was difficult. We knew we were satisfied, but there and right in front of us were platefuls of gâteaux and trifle. Food we had not seen or been near for months.

You talked it through with Judy, about the power struggle,

the fact that one part of us wants to eat and the other part wants to stop. I often feel that tug-of-war, when I want to eat and I know I should not. Usually in such a power struggle somebody wins, and somebody loses. There is no win or lose in this case. There is a question to ask though, 'Am I hungry?' and if I am I will eat something. If not, I need to do something different.

I asked Louise if I could take some of the cheese she had brought home with me. Then I got up from the table and walked around while those who were still hungry kept on eating.

I felt calm, and the next exercise made it even easier to leave my food behind. We were to pretend that we were five or six years old, and we had come to a 'play with your food' party. It was hilarious; at our table people started off cautiously by making designs and patterns in their food. As we got into the spirit of it, the fun really began. The lasagne which minutes before looked so delicious was rolled into a ball and sent to swim in a river of red wine. Carrots became noses on faces of mashed main course and garlic bread was a missile to hit any target which took our fancy. I screamed with laughter as Joy built a celery penis held up between two potato testicles; and I loved squelching trifle and tiramisu between my fingers. The food totally lost its attraction, after all, who wants to eat mud and cold potato faces?

I felt sad when I saw Dorothy cry so much, she said she was always punished when she was a child for playing with her food. The memories of my own childhood came spinning in as she spoke.

I was amazed at how many people found the next exercise so difficult. I did not, I marched up to that dustbin and chuckled as I scraped the food off my plate. What a waste, I heard somebody mutter. Yes, it was a waste, but I have never understood how I can help a starving child in Africa by finishing all the food on my plate. I have never, ever understood that logic. If I eat when I am not hungry *then* I am wasting food; my body does not require the food so it will turn it into fat. I do not need a fat store any more because I am lucky enough to be able to buy more food tomorrow. If I finish food when I am not hungry, and then I gain weight, how is that going to help a starving child anywhere? Starving myself is not the answer, eating and criticizing myself for eating and trying to diet uses up my energy, and I want it back.

After tonight's meal, I am going to waste less food, because I am going to prepare less. If I am eating anything, anywhere, and my inner voice says enough, I will stop. That is going to be the only issue.

I am quite sleepy now so I will end here, and I will see you next week . . .

Love, Norma

Conscious Eating

Eating like a naturally slim person requires lots of practice. You will not be able to do it perfectly overnight. While you are learning your new habits you need to unlearn years of old habits. Take it gradually, one step at a time. Always be kind to yourself, and when you make a mistake, treat it as a learning experience, remind yourself that you can learn from your mistakes. You will learn gradually: you may find that you take three steps forward and then two steps back. But one day you will realize you are eating like a naturally slim person without even thinking about it.

I know that you will want to overcome your eating problem as quickly as possible. It took years and years for you to end up in the destructive relationship with food that you have right now, so step by step we need to change the old and bring in a new relationship. The way to begin is to practise eating consciously. Experiment with giving up watching television while you are eating one week, and then the next week practise eating only off a plate. Make the changes slowly, one by one, and in the way that best suits your understanding and lifestyle. One day you may eat slowly and put your knife and fork down between bites, but the next you may totally forget about it. On the day you do remember, pat yourself on the back and say well done, well done. On the day you forget be reflective, ask yourself what you were feeling and why you forgot to take care of yourself. Never, ever criticize yourself, it gets you nowhere.

The Eating Directions

You may find the following summary of what we have discussed so far helpful. In the workshops, I call them the eating directions.

- Eat only when you are hungry. Always check when you want to eat that this is genuine body hunger and not mouth hunger.
  When you are hungry, give your hunger level a number. Aim to eat when you are moderately hungry, at number 3, and stop at 5, when you are satisfied.
- When you are hungry, eat exactly what you feel like eating. Ask yourself, if you had total freedom of choice, what would perfectly satisfy your hunger NOW! Go through various options: sweet or savoury, hot or cold, solid or liquid, crunchy or creamy or a combination of these. As you get to know your favourite foods, ensure that you always have a good supply of these.
- Once you have found out what is available, choose the closest possible to your needs. Decide approximately on quantity. It is an important part of the process to estimate the amount of food you feel you need. Finer adjustments can be made while you are eating.
- Be your own guest. Sit down, put your food on a plate and eat in a nice environment.

- Eat without distraction so that you concentrate on stopping when you are satisfied. Be aware of your hunger level changing and look out for taste changes to signal when you are satisfied.
- Enjoy, taste, savour every mouthful. Eat your best food first.
- Eat slowly.
- Stop when you are satisfied.

One of the most important things to remember about the Weigh Ahead eating directions is that they are just guidelines. They are not rules! When you decided to stop dieting, you stopped following other people's rules and stopped handing over control to an expert or a diet. I have merely suggested principles which made it easier for me when I decided to live like a naturally slim person. They have worked for many others. But everyone is different: some of them may not work for you. Test them out, question each eating direction and then choose what works for you. You may discover directions of your own. The important thing is not to create rigidity and rules. You know yourself all too well by now: rules are there for you to break. If you are too rigid in what you allow yourself, you will rebel against your rules, and you will find yourself in the old self-destructive behaviour. Please be flexible, be kind to yourself, and forgive yourself for any lapses. I know you can do it: soon, like me, you will be eating like a naturally slim person.

When you learn to ride a bicycle for the first time, you start off being unconsciously unskilled: not only are you inexperienced and unskilled at riding the bike, but you are not even aware of what you need to know to get the hang of it. After your first lesson, you become consciously unskilled: you now know you need to keep your balance, but you still don't always manage to keep yourself from falling off. With some practice, and by concentrating on all the steps you have been taught, you eventually manage to cycle to your destination without falling off: you have become consciously skilled. After you have been cycling every day for some weeks, you no longer need to

THE NATURALLY SLIM EATING FLOW CHART

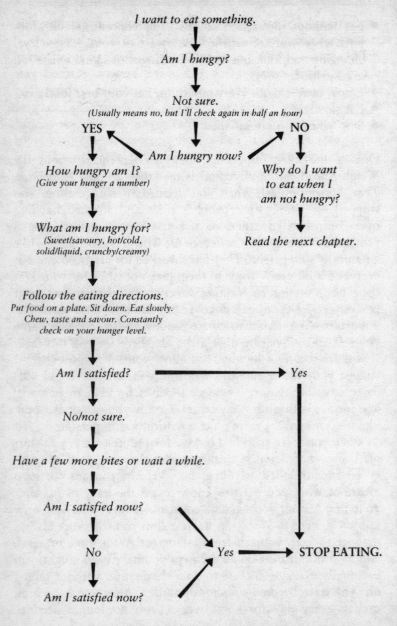

- Eat without distraction so that you concentrate on stopping when you are satisfied. Be aware of your hunger level changing and look out for taste changes to signal when you are satisfied.
- Enjoy, taste, savour every mouthful. Eat your best food first.
- Eat slowly.
- Stop when you are satisfied.

One of the most important things to remember about the Weigh Ahead eating directions is that they are just guidelines. They are not rules! When you decided to stop dieting, you stopped following other people's rules and stopped handing over control to an expert or a diet. I have merely suggested principles which made it easier for me when I decided to live like a naturally slim person. They have worked for many others. But everyone is different: some of them may not work for you. Test them out, question each eating direction and then choose what works for you. You may discover directions of your own. The important thing is not to create rigidity and rules. You know yourself all too well by now: rules are there for you to break. If you are too rigid in what you allow yourself, you will rebel against your rules, and you will find yourself in the old self-destructive behaviour. Please be flexible, be kind to yourself, and forgive yourself for any lapses. I know you can do it: soon, like me, you will be eating like a naturally slim person.

When you learn to ride a bicycle for the first time, you start off being unconsciously unskilled: not only are you inexperienced and unskilled at riding the bike, but you are not even aware of what you need to know to get the hang of it. After your first lesson, you become consciously unskilled: you now know you need to keep your balance, but you still don't always manage to keep yourself from falling off. With some practice, and by concentrating on all the steps you have been taught, you eventually manage to cycle to your destination without falling off: you have become consciously skilled. After you have been cycling every day for some weeks, you no longer need to

THE NATURALLY SLIM EATING FLOW CHART

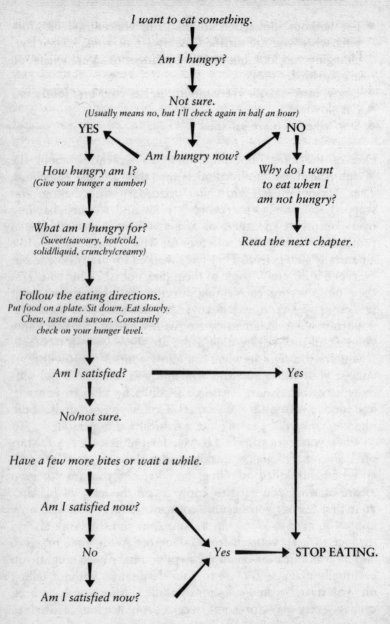

I want to eat something.

Am I hungry?

Not sure.
(Usually means no, but I'll check again in half an hour)

YES   *Am I hungry now?*   **NO**

How hungry am I?
(Give your hunger a number)

Why do I want to eat when I am not hungry?

What am I hungry for?
(Sweet/savoury, hot/cold, solid/liquid, crunchy/creamy)

Read the next chapter.

Follow the eating directions.
Put food on a plate. Sit down. Eat slowly.
Chew, taste and savour. Constantly
check on your hunger level.

Am I satisfied? ——→ *Yes*

No/not sure.

Have a few more bites or wait a while.

Am I satisfied now?

No

Am I satisfied now?

Yes ——→ **STOP EATING.**

concentrate on what you are doing to retain your balance; this means you are now unconsciously skilled at riding a bike.

Perhaps when you began reading this book you had never thought about eating when you were hungry. Rather, you ate in response to a whole raft of suppressed feelings that had nothing to do with your hunger. You could not control your behaviour around food, because you did not understand the link between your eating and your emotions. You were unconsciously unskilled. After reading the first few chapters of this book, you learnt how naturally slim people eat, but it was very difficult for you to apply that knowledge to your own life. You were consciously unskilled, and you still lapsed back into your old habits although you recognized what you were doing and knew it made you miserable. When the time comes that for most of the time you manage to eat only when you are hungry, and find other ways of dealing with painful feelings, you will have passed into the third stage and will have become consciously skilled. As the days pass and you continue to eat only when you are hungry, you will eventually reach a point when you are doing it instinctively most of the time, without even thinking about it. This is your goal; to become unconsciously skilled, just like any other naturally slim person.

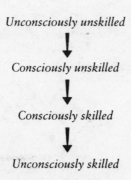

Unconsciously unskilled

↓

Consciously unskilled

↓

Consciously skilled

↓

Unconsciously skilled

There are still great difficulties to overcome. In my workshops, in the session after I have explained the eating directions, it is almost inevitable that someone will burst out angrily, 'Cherie, all this is all very well, but why do I still want to eat when I am not hungry?' If you still want to eat when you are not hungry, you need to delve deeper into the forces that drive you, as I shall explain in the next chapter.

PART 2

3

If I'm Not Hungry, Why Do I Keep Wanting to Eat?

'Eating when I was hungry sounded good, but the best part about food was eating when I wasn't hungry. Food was the glue that held my life together between hungers.'

GENEEN ROTH

After practising the eating directions for a week, Joyce returned to the workshop and burst out in angry tears: 'Cherie, it all started out so wonderfully, I have managed to listen to my hunger for the first time in years. I enjoy eating and I don't feel bloated. But why do I feel all out of sorts? I'm weepy, I'm angry, I don't know what to do, this is not like me at all.'

On the surface, eating like a slim person sounds so easy, doesn't it? Eat when you are hungry, eat exactly what you want and stop when you are satisfied. But, as you can see, there are

still a lot of pages left in this book, because there is still a lot
of work to be done. Although we can learn to eat like naturally slim people, there is still a *big difference* between naturally
slim people and compulsive eaters. Naturally slim people only
want to eat when they are hungry. Compulsive eaters want to
eat, and eat and then eat some more, even when they are not
hungry.

To compulsive eaters, food has been invested with magic
and mystique. For them food represents comfort, friendship
and love. When you take the surplus food away from a
compulsive eater she is left with a vacuum, a wide gaping
hole that she believes only food can fill. She cannot stop eating
compulsively until she has identified the hole, and learned to fill
it, with something other than food.

Dear Cherie,
I think about food all the time. I use food to calm me down
and to perk me up. I think of food when I wake up and when
I go to sleep. When I am not thinking of food I am dreaming
about losing weight, I would so love to lose weight! I want to
wear jeans, I want to slink into the room in a low cut black
evening gown. I want to be thin.

I want to lose weight and if I eat only when I am hungry
then I can do that. But the big problem is that I get a crazy
all-consuming hunger when I am not hungry. On a logical level
it all sounds easy; if I go on a diet, if I do all the right things
and I eat less then I know I will lose weight. If I am honest,
though, it feels as if logic and common sense play no part in
this no-win situation. I want to eat all the time and I also want
to be thinner.

I have a good job, a wonderful husband, and two bright
lovely children. I regularly see my friends, and I have a lovely
life. But there is a demon that lives with me, Cherie. When I
pinch my thighs in the morning, the fat bulges at me. When
I get dressed my mirror shouts, 'You fat cow, get thinner.' I
know I am fat, but when there is space in the day and I am

there and food is there you cannot keep the two of us apart. Food is my magnet and it pulls me with an irresistible force. I want to get thinner. I can't stop eating.

Please help. In the magazine article about you it says that you managed to lose weight without dieting, can you please tell me how you managed to do that, how do you spend your days without overeating?

Love, June

I get so many letters and meet so many people who are in the same situation as June, the same seemingly hopeless tug-of-war. They want to lose weight, but they cannot stop overeating. I can only help June if she is willing to look at why she has this overwhelming desire to eat when she is not hungry, only if she is willing to admit that she is a compulsive eater, and that that is a serious problem which needs to be addressed.

I used to be terrified to be at home on my own for any period of time because I knew that being at home meant I would overeat. Now I live and work at home. As I have been writing this book I have spent hours alone with a word processor. Sometimes the words flow freely and easily and the pages fly out, and at other times each paragraph takes three hours, and each word feels as if it is stuck in mud. At times like these it is especially difficult; the kitchen is always there, the food continues to beckon. Every time I stop working I have the choice: to eat something or not to eat something. If I had been doing this book eight years ago I would have gained twenty pounds; this time I may have gained a pound or two. To answer June's question, how I have done that? How have I spent my days without overeating?

The answer is that I have turned the urge to eat when I am not hungry into a valuable warning system, an alarm bell that tells me that I need something. I know that I am a compulsive eater, and I know that if I want to eat when I am not hungry, then something is wrong. Every single time I want to eat when I am not hungry I ask myself this question: 'Cherie, why, why

do you want to eat if you are not hungry? Is something wrong?'
Then I have a little conversation with myself so that I can seek
out the reason, and look for the feeling that is hidden behind
my desire for food.

Eight years ago the only way I knew to deal with my feelings
was to go into the kitchen and eat something. Today I know
that if I want to eat when I am not hungry I need to take care
of myself. Maybe I need a walk, or to talk with somebody,
maybe I am scared or anxious or bored or I need a cry. The
more I have learnt to listen to my feelings, the needs hidden
behind my desire to eat when I am not hungry, the easier it
has become to eat only when I am hungry.

Sometimes it is easy to do something about the hidden feeling,
and sometimes it is really difficult. Sometimes I am in the kitchen
with both hands in the biscuit tin and two biscuits in my mouth
before I remember that I am not hungry. At other times I know
I am not hungry, but the urge to eat is so all-consuming and
overwhelming that I eat anyway. But mostly I have learnt to
remain in touch with my feelings and be aware of what is
happening inside me. When the desire to eat comes, and I am
not hungry, I can catch it, deflect it, and try to give myself
what I really need.

You too can turn your problem, which is the urge to eat
when you are not hungry, into your solution. Your urge to
overeat can be the friend you need, the one who tells you that
you need to pay attention to yourself. Instead of fighting against
the urge to eat you can teach yourself to use it as a way to get
to know yourself.

We did not simply wake up one day with a problem with food,
it took years. Over those years we have *learned* to behave in a
certain way, as if a computer programme has been written into
our heads, a programme that translates all our feelings and needs
– our boredom, our excitement, our anger, our loneliness, our
happiness, our sadness or our anxiety – into the same answer.
Eat something.

We feel sad and the programme says: eat something.

We have an argument and the programme says: eat something.

We finish the housework, the programme says: eat something.

We feel happy, angry, drained.

We have to cope with a crisis.

We have to work late.

We are having a break at work.

We have to do something we don't want to do.

The programme is stuck in the same place: whatever we do, think, or feel, we get the same message: eat something, eat something, eat something.

I was at the train station the other day. Next to me was a mother with a baby and a young child. The mother had a bottle and a packet of sweets, and every time the baby made any noise whatsoever she shoved the bottle in its mouth, and every time the young child spoke, asked a question or tried to point out something, the mother's reaction was the same: she offered a sweet. That is the programming I mean. If that happens every day, those two children will grow up having learned to answer all needs with food.

Perhaps you were lucky enough to eat naturally when you were a child, and the only time you ate when you were not hungry was when there was an extra special treat to eat. But then you went on that first diet. In Chapter 1 I outlined how years of dieting and weight-watching caused an ever-increasing obsession with food and with your weight; how by making certain foods forbidden we want them even more, how we put off our lives until we got thin, how our self-esteem became wrapped up in what we weighed, and how the horrible cycle of dieting and bingeing made our lives a nightmare. We have wrapped ourselves in the problem like the layers of an onion, trapping us, enclosing us, making us cry.

If you have been obsessed with your weight for years, you need to peel away those layers one by one, examining each layer as you peel it away. The rest of this book is about the journey you will need to take to recover from your compulsive eating.

I have divided that journey into the following steps:

First step: Discovering the links between your eating and your emotions (Chapter 4).
Second step: Learning to identify and express your feelings (Chapters 5 and 6).
Third step: Learning to accept yourself (Chapter 7).
Fourth step: Rediscovering your body (Chapter 8).
Fifth step: Nourishing yourself without using food (Chapter 9).
Sixth step: The root of the problem: Confronting your past history (Chapter 10).

4

A Banquet of Fear, Excitement and Sadness: Discovering the Links between Eating and Your Emotions

'Now, piece by piece, we come to see how food has ceased to be a purely inanimate object . . .'

KIM CHERNIN

If my television set was not working I would call a repair man in to fix it. Before he began doing any actual repair work, he would have to find the fault. So too with our eating. Before we can stop overeating we need to find out the fault, that is, we need to pinpoint the exact foods, situations and feeling which cause us to overeat. An easy way to do that is through filling in a food chart. Record every time you eat anything – what you ate, where you were, what you were thinking, how you felt, how you felt afterwards. Perhaps in your past dieting days you filled in such a chart in order to see if you were following a diet correctly, and hated it. This is different. It is an invaluable tool for discovering why you eat when you are not hungry; it will provide a map to the situations, foods, thoughts and feelings that trigger you to eat. I suggest that you fill it in for a week. Be careful not to use your chart as a whip with which to punish yourself with for overeating – this is an exercise to learn from, not to berate yourself with. Once you have identified when you overeat you can begin to plan ways of dealing with it.

The first column is to record the time of the day you ate. The next column will record whether you were hungry or not. In the third column write down what you ate, and in the one after that, fill in how and where you ate it. For example: 'I ate it quickly, standing in the kitchen,' or 'I put the biscuits into my pocket and broke off little pieces to sneak into my mouth when nobody was looking!' or 'I ate slowly, sitting down at the table.'

Column five asks what you were thinking and feeling before eating, and column 6 records how you felt after eating. Because the word feel has so many meanings, let me explain what I mean by it.

A *feeling* usually begins with the words 'I am' or 'I feel'; for example – I feel sad, I am happy, I feel irritated, angry, bored, lonely, excited. However, 'I feel' is also used in a different way, which can cause confusion. 'I feel that there is going to be a change of government' is actually an opinion, not a feeling. 'I feel that he is dishonest' is a judgement, not a feeling. When you begin a statement with 'I feel that . . .', where you could just as easily say 'I believe that' or 'I think that', it is usually not a feeling, but rather a thought, opinion or judgement which reflects your beliefs.

It is also important to remember to distinguish between physical feelings, sensations in your body, and your emotions. Although you use 'I feel hungry' to describe the bodily sensation of hunger, hunger is not an emotion like sadness, anger and anxiety. You feel the physical sensation of hunger in your body like you feel cold, tired, dizzy or a cramp in your left foot.

As you look at your chart, see if you can identify patterns.

Which feelings always send you straight to the fridge? Boredom? Anger? Anxiety? Pain?

Which situations do you always cope with by overeating? Tea-time with the children? Family arguments? Stress at work? Coming into an empty house? Being on holiday?

What time of the day or day of the week is particularly difficult? Do you for example always overeat on a Sunday, when the usual routine of the week is changed? Is ten o'clock at night a regular overeating time for you? Or when you come home from work? Or when you watch TV?

What particular foods do you regularly overeat on? Chocolate? Crisps? Bread? Cheese?

Suzy came back to the group after filling in her chart for two weeks. 'It was amazing,' she said. 'I realize I am dreadfully confused. I have confused the word hunger with every other feeling or excuse under the sun. There it was, written in black and white, just how often I was eating when I was not hungry. I ate when I was sad, happy, excited, angry, stressed, tired, not tired, lonely, bored, frustrated. Every feeling meant hungry. It was also interesting to see *when* I eat: I seem to eat to fill the gap between everything I do. The gap between arriving home from work, and being at home. The gap between changing from one activity to another. If I was watching television I ate in the commercial breaks, and between programmes.'

Rachel joined in and said, 'I found that late at night when I was home alone, especially Sunday nights, were a difficult time for me, and also that giving dinner parties were a disaster area. While I was cooking I got really anxious, and I "tasted" so much food it was the equivalent of an extra guest's portion. When my guests left I cleared away more food into my stomach. And I know why: I was tired, I was angry at having to do the washing up, and I was furious at myself for overeating.'

The food chart example on page 134–35 is from Pat, who is a PA in a large company and has two children. From her chart

Pat identified two situations in which she always felt compelled to eat when she was not hungry:

(a) When she was giving the children tea she became a vacuum-cleaner eater. She would eat while she was cooking, then she would finish the children's leftovers, before struggling to eat a meal with her husband later.
(b) Late at night, while she was watching television, food would constantly beckon her into the kitchen.

Once she was aware of this pattern, Pat worked out some new strategies.

(a) Pat said that when she was preparing the children's tea she felt really stressed. She was tired, the children were needy, and it was as if she was being pulled in a hundred different directions at once. Eating as a way to cope with all this was making her feel worse. She spoke to a counsellor and discovered that if she dealt with her anxiety — took deep breaths, did one thing at a time, set out something definite for the children to do — she ate a lot less.
(b) In the evening, watching TV, Pat found herself eating for a variety of feelings. Her husband belonged to a Rotary club and was at a meeting once a week, and he often worked late at night. She resented the fact that she was stuck at home alone, and felt bored and lonely, so she would eat to switch off her feelings. Once she had identified her feelings she made plans to deal with them. She confronted her husband and he agreed to work at home some evenings. For the times she was at home alone, she made a list of ways to distract herself from eating: phone a friend, invite a friend over, write in her journal, arrange a babysitter for the nights John was at Rotary and go to her health club, clean out a drawer, give herself a manicure, have a long bath, learn to be with herself and her feelings, go to bed early.

What problems and feelings are *you* eating away?

Lucy found that she would hang around the kitchen late at night, on the pretext that she was preparing food for the next day. She dragged out the task for as long as possible. What she was actually doing was hoping that by the time she got to bed her husband would be asleep. She had been trying to avoid sex with him for years. In her chart the entry read: '11 p.m., not hungry, feeling anxious. Ate a biscuit, some cold cottage pie, a banana, three little Mars bars. I ate everything walking around in the kitchen, still anxious, listening for sounds from upstairs. After eating I felt unhappy: writing this chart made me realize that I am eating my anxiety away at night because I don't want to get into bed with my husband.'

When Marcus had woken up that morning he had dived into the kitchen to eat three pieces of toast and a huge bowl of cereal. When the tea trolley came around at work, he ordered a large doughnut with his tea. It was only mid-bite through the doughnut that he remembered to ask himself what he was doing, why he was eating so much. The answer was right there, staring him in the face. Yesterday, he had been told to report at 5.00 today to 'the den'. This was the nickname that employees had given his boss's office. He had no idea what the meeting was about and he was scared, no, more than scared – he was terrified. For all he knew he was about to be fired. Then he realized that he always had the urge to nibble when he thought about his boss, and it dawned on him that he felt deeply insecure about his position in the firm. Once Marcus was aware of his anxiety, he decided he had nothing to lose by asking his boss for a job review, an assessment of his effectiveness. At least he would know where he stood.

Pamela's chart got very crowded two or three times a week – during and after her mother called. Her telephone is in the kitchen, and as soon as they started talking Pam's hand would reach for the chocolate and she would nibble compulsively right through the conversation. When the conversation was over she would take whole handfuls of food and shovel them in. It was to cover up her feelings – her mother still commented and judged everything that she did or said. She felt compelled to tell her mother everything and ask for advice, just like a four-year-old child. She coped with all the feelings that went with that – her hurt, her anger, her resentment – by eating. Once Pam realized this she could begin to work on the real problem – her relationship with her mother.

On Mondays, Tuesdays, and Wednesdays Karen does training for sales staff. She spends her whole day running workshops. On her food chart she noticed that she is not usually hungry at lunch-time but she always eats something. She mentioned this one evening during her Weigh Ahead course and I asked her how she usually felt during lunch-time. She thought about it for a while and then realized that she felt a mixture of tiredness and loneliness. She kept herself separate from the group because she was the group leader and she answered her feelings and the need to reward herself for a hard morning's work by eating something. The group suggested some other ways Karen could spend her lunch hour and feel rewarded and rested: go for a walk, buy a magazine and read it, go shopping, arrange to meet a friend for a talk, make an appointment at the hairdresser, take a Walkman or sit in the car and listen to Cherie's relaxation tape.

After discussing the food chart in the Weigh Ahead group, a version of the following question often crops up: 'Isn't this back to standard diet advice, Cherie? We had to fill in charts and distract ourselves from food by going to the hairdresser, when we were dieting. We get this kind of advice from magazines.'

Diets are about deprivation, about not trusting yourself, about distracting yourself from food. This programme is about identifying and fulfilling your real needs. You need to short-circuit the programme which sends you to food when you are not hungry and replace it with a new programme, which will send you to the place you really need to be. When you are tired, rest. If you are lonely, phone someone or invite a friend round. When you are angry, express your anger and address the situation which is causing it. Do something instead of eating something.

Learning to address and answer your real needs can be much more difficult than using food: when you are lonely it can be easier to eat chocolate than to reach out to others and risk being rejected. When you are angry with your husband it may be easier to bury your anger in the fridge instead of confronting him with your feelings and causing a row. When you are depressed you will really miss the momentary lift that food gives you. But unless you address the underlying problem, it will not go away. A boring job is going to stay boring no matter how many Mars bars you eat. A bad relationship will not change if every time you have an argument you make cheesecake the solution.

I know, it's difficult to break the habits of a lifetime. You have been reaching for a packet of crisps when you have to do the ironing for years. You have sought the hug you need in a doughnut for so long now that you don't even know you are doing it. If you take the time and trouble to listen to how you are really feeling, to give yourself what you really need, then you will stop wanting to eat when you are not hungry.

Here is another question course participants often ask me: 'Surely all this thinking about eating, and whether I'm hungry or not, and why I'm overeating, is encouraging my obsession with food?'

I agree that in the beginning you do have to spend a lot of time thinking about your eating. But you are giving it *positive*, constructive attention so that you can learn from it, which is very different from the negative obsessing about food and your weight which leads you nowhere.

EXAMPLE OF FOOD CHART (PAT)

WHEN	HUNGRY	WHAT	HOW AND WHERE	THOUGHTS AND FEELINGS	
				BEFORE EATING	AFTER EATING
8am	Yes	All-Bran	Sat down	Calm and on time today	Full of energy
10am	No	Black coffee	Desk	Upset – John said he would be home late	Still upset – third time this week
1pm	Yes	Baked potato Cottage cheese	Ate very fast in canteen	Lots of work to do – feel anxious	Thought that everyone noticed how fast I'm eating
5.30pm	Yes	Apple Black coffee	Sat with Kim while she did her homework	No cooking – taking the kids for a pizza	Happy
6.30pm	Yes	Tuna salad Bite of pizza	Italian restaurant Ate slowly	Enjoyed myself	Drained and so much to do
10–12pm	No	Biscuit Another biscuit Packet of crisps	Watching TV	Bored waiting for John to return home	Angry with myself

WHEN	HUNGRY	WHAT	HOW AND WHERE	THOUGHTS AND FEELINGS BEFORE EATING	THOUGHTS AND FEELINGS AFTER EATING
8am	Yes	All-Bran	Standing in kitchen	Rushing getting everybody ready to leave	Stressed
10am	Slightly	Tea and biscuit	At desk	Excited about new project	Felt a bit guilty about biscuit
1pm	Yes	Chicken salad sandwich Diet Coke	Park Read newspaper	Motivated Full of energy	Thinking about what to cook tonight
5.30pm	No	Cheese cracker Taste of stew	In kitchen while cooking. Ate with fingers all out of pot	Tired	Stressed – kids, homework and I just ate
7pm	No	Stew, rice Ice-cream	Family dinner	Feel fat	I will always be fat – feel awful
10pm	Slightly	Low-cal chocolate drink Oat cake	In bed	Tired Feel fat	Wish I was thin – I'll be good tomorrow

5

Talking to Yourself: Learning to Identify and Express Your Feelings

'Don't let some dumb little kid ruin the rest of your life.'

ALVYN M. FREED

'Praise is the best diet for us after all.'

REVD SYDNEY SMITH

Wednesday Night, Session Three, Weigh Ahead Programme

Cherie: What feelings do you have in your body when you know you need to cry? Where exactly do you feel emotional pain?

Answers from the Group: Lump in my throat. Choking feeling in my neck. Knife-like pain in the centre of my chest. Shoulders feel paralysed.

Cherie: What foods do you eat when you feel a lump in your throat, pain in your chest and paralysed shoulders?
Group: Hot sweet tea, creamy food, white bread, mashed potatoes and gravy. Soup.

Cherie: Where in your body do you feel anger; how do you know you are really cross about something?
Group: I feel like I want to explode, I feel tension right across my shoulders and in my chest. I feel anger in my throat, neck. I feel it in my head.

Cherie: What foods do you eat when you are angry?
Group: Carrots and crunchy foods, like toast, apples, peanuts, crisps and curries.

Cherie: Where in your body do you feel anxiety?
Group: I feel a pressure in my head. In my stomach, butterflies in my stomach, sweaty palms, whole body feels shaky.

Cherie: And what do you want to eat when you are anxious?
Group: Anything that will calm me down, chocolate, crisps, biscuits, cheese, hot milky drinks.

Cherie: Where in your body do you feel sexual?
Group: All over, in my groin, my breasts, my mouth, my stomach.

Cherie: What do you eat when you feel sexy?
Group: Smooth and creamy, ice-cream, chocolate, peanut butter. I take a Toblerone to bed.

Cherie: So where in your body do you feel hunger?
Group: Silence. Shrugs. Don't know. Umm, my stomach? I'm not sure. Perhaps my throat?

Isn't that revealing? A roomful of intelligent, articulate people

showed that none of them was quite sure how to differentiate
hunger from all their other feelings. Hunger is a physical sensation; sadness, anxiety, anger, and boredom are feelings. Hunger
is the only feeling that needs to be answered with food. When
we answer any of our other feelings with food, we lose touch
with our feelings, we feel miserable without knowing why, and
we get fat.

As Joanne drove into her driveway she heard a thud followed
by a loud scratching noise and her heart sank to her knees as
she realized that she had driven her new car into the concrete
gatepost. She burst out crying, and felt as helpless as a child.
Then she began to shout at herself: 'Why weren't you more
careful, you stupid idiot, you've really done it now, if you paid
a bit more attention you would not drive like an imbecile. You
are stupid, stupid, stupid!' When she had calmed down, she went
inside the house, phoned her insurance company, then made an
appointment at the garage to have the damage assessed.

An outsider who was watching Joanne would have noticed
that during this incident her behaviour went through three very
different stages. Dr Eric Berne, the originator of Transactional
Analysis, was the first person to suggest that all of us think,
behave and feel in three very different ways. He called these
three different ways of being our Parent, Adult and Child Ego
states.

When we were little children we were small, wonderful,
wild and powerless. Our parents imposed rules, discipline and
punishment on us; but they were also the source of cuddles,
praise and comfort.

When we grew up, these aspects of our upbringing became
absorbed into our personality, and inside each of us there is a
child, a critical parent and a nurturing parent, as well as the
sensible adult we have learned to be. These different selves take
turns to direct our actions. When Joanne crashed into the gatepost she first of all became childlike, she cried and felt helpless
and miserable – this means that her child self was dominant at
that particular moment. When she shouted at herself she was in

her critical parent self, and when she was logically organizing her insurance and repair, her adult self was in charge.

The parent self has two sides, a critical side and a nurturing side. Most compulsive eaters talk to themselves in a very critical way all day. This voice we use is the side of our self we can call the critical parent or the inner critic. The critical parent will always use words like should, could, must, will, shut up, idiot, fat pig. 'No, you are not allowed to eat that.' 'You must lose some weight.' 'You stupid idiot, you always mess things up.' 'Someone with a bit of brain would have done it this way.' 'You are absolutely useless, you will never be anything.' When you notice yourself talking like this you know that you are 'coming on parent'.

The nurturing parent, on the other hand, will be kind and warm and caring. For some of us she/he is a distant memory of the safest part of our own childhood.

'Take a coat, honey, it's cold out there.' 'I love you. Are you all right?' 'You are so tired, why don't you have a rest?' 'Well done, you really did that well.' 'There is absolutely nothing wrong with you.' This is the part of ourselves that nurtures our children and the people we love. We would feel much better if we spoke to ourselves with our nurturing instead of our critical parent all day, but many of us find that very difficult indeed.

The child self, which nowadays is often referred to as the inner child, also has many parts. When you were a baby and you were cuddled you felt good and loved, and you laughed and squealed. When you were sore or lonely you felt sad and cried, or you got angry and let everybody around you know by shouting and throwing a temper tantrum. You were born with the ability to feel all sorts of emotions – anger, happiness, frustration, excitement – and to express them physically. As you have grown you have not lost the ability to feel all these feelings, but the ability to express them has often been lost. Words and behaviours from your child are usually as a result of these feelings. Words your child might use: 'I want,' 'I feel,'

'Nobody loves me.' 'I feel sad/scared/lonely/angry.' 'I want it now!' 'I wish.' 'I hope.' 'I want to have fun.'

Think about the last time you really enjoyed yourself. What were you feeling? The chances are you were happy, excited, joyful, contented or a mixture of these. Perhaps you felt like skipping or jumping for joy. This part of your child, with all your unharnessed feelings running free, is your natural child. As we grew, however, we were forced to adapt and to conform to society. We had to learn not to cross a busy street, only to pee in the toilet, to sit quietly in class even if we were bored. Some children adapt in a 'passive' way, that is, they do everything that is expected of them, they do things to please their parents and other adults. Other children are more rebellious. Have you ever noticed that when you say to a child 'No, don't do that! the child can become defiant and actually wants to do the direct opposite of what they have been told? This is also part of our child, the rebellious adapted child.

Rebellious, defiant child. If you think about it, that is exactly what the child inside us has grown to be over the years of dieting. As we sat with grilled chicken and steamed cabbage and watched as others tucked into pies and puddings our child was getting more and more rebellious and defiant. She was actually becoming more and more determined to have food we were not allowed. Each and every time we said no to foods we really wanted, each and every time we went hungry the defiance grew. And it is this defiant rebellious child who overeats, and binges, and causes the eating havoc in our lives.

You may wonder why I am telling you all this, but if there ever was a magic wand to wave over our eating problems this is it. You see, when you go on a diet, you are creating a war inside yourself. Your critical parent is shouting and yelling about how fat and disgusting you are, and your rebellious child is saying I need to eat nice things, I am sick of this deprivation, if you make me diet I'll show you next time there is nice food around I am gonna eat it all!!! You need to bring a negotiator into this tug-of-war, someone who can step in, listen to both sides of the argument and negotiate a settlement. This conciliator exists within you as well, and she is called your adult.

Our adult tries to deal with the present – behaviours, thoughts and feelings in the here and now. Our adult is concerned with facts, she is precise, she makes sense and sees things the way they really are. Your adult does not make judgements about your behaviour. She stays neutral and logical. Words your adult might say: 'It is,' 'I think,' 'Are you hungry?' 'What are the facts?' 'My first choice is . . .' 'How far have you got in solving the problem?' 'I think that we should try the left turn.'

Talking to your Inner Child

Now that you know about your inner child, adult and parent, I am going to suggest a method for getting in touch with your real feelings which you may at first find odd, but which gets much more comfortable with practice. Remember the eating directions? If I ask myself, 'Am I hungry?' and the answer is no, what I do is start a conversation with my inner child to find out what is wrong.

Do you think only crazy people talk to themselves? Don't worry, you don't have to talk to yourself out loud and in public. But if you ask your child what is wrong and listen to the answer, you will begin to understand your own behaviour. Sometimes your child will say she is eating in defiance because there is illegal food around and she is sick of carrot sticks. At other times, your child will be eating as a result of a feeling, because she has learnt that food can suppress all uncomfortable feelings.

I began eating compulsively when I was three years old. That was the way I survived my childhood. When I want to eat and I know I am not hungry, I have a conversation with my Child. I call her Little Cherie, and I often think of her as a three-year-old. This vulnerable, precious part of myself needs to be looked after, to be loved, and I am the only person available to do that.

I was at home with a sore back. For four days I had been lying flat on my back, legs up, head down. Now I was up again but still could not leave the house or drive. I watched TV, cleared my desk, and then heard a little voice say: 'Let's finish off the cake in the tin.' So I had a conversation with that little voice in my head:

Cherie: Are you hungry?
Little Cherie: No.
Cherie: Then why do you want to eat?
Little Cherie: Well, what else is there to do?
Cherie: Are you bored?
Little Cherie: I guess so.
Cherie: I know we have been stuck in this house for days, but I don't want you to eat when you are not hungry. How about we do something else instead. We could phone someone, or we could take out the paints and brushes, or we could have a bath.
Little Cherie: Let's paint. And can we eat cake when I am hungry.
Cherie: Of course, if you still want it then.

Talking to your inner child takes practice. Your defiant child is going to want to eat, and you have to talk her out of it. Don't try to win a battle, but rather aim to negotiate a settlement. Try to talk in your nurturing parent voice, and tell your critical parent to make herself scarce.

Penny was at the service station and she found herself looking at the rows of chocolate.

Penny: Are you hungry?
Little Penny: No, but I want a chocolate.
Penny: Why do you want to eat when you are not hungry?
Little Penny: I am fed up!!! I'm tired and I don't feel like all the traffic on the way home.

Penny: I hear that you are tired and angry, but how will having a chocolate help?

Little Penny: Well, I will forget about being tired while I am eating it!!!

Penny: I really don't want you to have a chocolate for tiredness and frustration; how about if we go into a café, read the newspaper and have a hot drink, and drive home when there is less traffic.

Little Penny: No, I'd rather have the chocolate, and go home.

Penny: I am so sorry that you feel the need to comfort yourself with chocolate – I really don't want to let you have it. How about we buy the chocolate for later but it will have to go in the boot until we get home. Then I'll play some really soothing music in the car, and I promise you if you are hungry for chocolate later, then you can eat the chocolate.

Little Penny: OK, and when we get home I want to relax and not rush around.

Penny: Fine.

In this conversation it is clear that Penny was firm, but also understanding, just like a nurturing person should be. She affirmed that Little Penny was tired and angry but she did not allow her to eat the chocolate. She gave her another option for dealing with her tiredness and frustration and she promised that she could eat the chocolate later if she still wanted it. In her former dieting days Penny would have felt a tug-of-war inside: eat–not eat–eat, and whatever side won she would have felt miserable. If she had given in to the temptation of chocolate, she would have hated herself, and if she hadn't, she would have felt deprived. In both cases, her tiredness and frustration would have gone unacknowledged.

Mary had gone out to a movie one evening and as she arrived home she realized that she wanted to eat even though she was not hungry.

Child Mary: I can't go to bed without eating *anything*.

Mary: Are you hungry?

Child Mary: No.

Mary: Why do you want to eat, then?

Child Mary: I'm scared, I feel so scared to go to bed without eating something.

Mary: You're scared, honey? Why?

Child Mary: It doesn't feel right, I feel as if I am leaving something behind that I really need.

Mary: I also know that you won't feel right if you eat when you are not hungry. I know, I'll make you a nice hot-water-bottle, and put on your warm fluffy pyjamas.

Child Mary: But will I be all right without eating something?

Mary: Of course you will, I'll take care of you, food cannot take care of you, you just got into bad habits of thinking that it does. Come on upstairs, you don't need to be scared, we'll cuddle into bed and get really warm.

Sometimes your defiant child is just going to win, she wants to eat and there is nothing you can do to talk her out of it. But there is no point in having a fight about it; try always to be kind to yourself, and muzzle your nagging critical parent. Sue was at a dinner party and half-way through dinner she got the signal that she was satisfied. She still wanted to carry on eating, though, so she asked her inner child why.

Sue: Why are you wanting to carry on eating?

Inner Sue: It's such nice food, and we never have food like this at home. And in any case there was cream in the soup so I have blown the calorie count anyway.

Sue: I agree the food is nice, but please remember I am not dieting any more and so you do not need to worry that I will deprive you of food in the future.

Inner Sue: I don't care, I want a second helping of this lamb stew, *and* I want dessert *and* I want cheese and biscuits, and you can't stop me.

Sue: You really want to overeat, and I really don't want you to.

Inner Sue: Well, I am going to *and you can't stop me*.

Sue: How are you feeling?

Inner Sue: What?

Sue: How are you feeling?

Inner Sue: Don't start with that feeling crap, I want to eat.

Sue: I am sorry that you are feeling so cross that you want to take that anger out on us by eating.

Inner Sue: I am angry, and I am frustrated. I am not enjoying being here. There are all these thin people, I am the only fat one. I am bored, I want to go home!!

Sue: I am sorry you feel fat and that you are bored, and eating is not going to solve anything.

Inner Sue: You cannot stop me, I will eat, I want to and I am going to.

Sue: I am sad that you need to eat, because of the way you are feeling. I am still going to be kind to you. I know in the past I criticized you every time you overate. Now I know you are eating because you are unhappy. I am working on and will find other ways to comfort you.

Inner Sue: (Eats.)

Sue: I am really sorry that you need to eat because you feel excluded and because you are bored. I am not angry, and we will continue to find other solutions for our overeating.

When you begin to dialogue with your inner child, feelings are bound to come flooding up – feelings you may not have been aware of for years. All children are born with the ability to express their feelings. They cry as soon as they feel discomfort or pain, stamp their feet and scream when they are angry, and they laugh out loud when they feel happy and joyful. But children are soon taught to control their feelings. From a very early age we are told things like don't cry, pull yourself together, don't shout, stop giggling, I'll give you something to cry about, don't be a baby. We become so much in control that we lose touch with ourselves, with what we really feel.

We pay a price to be so in control. Feelings are a form of energy, and in order to control our feelings we need to use up a greater amount of energy than that of the actual feeling.

THE NATURALLY SLIM HUNGER CHART

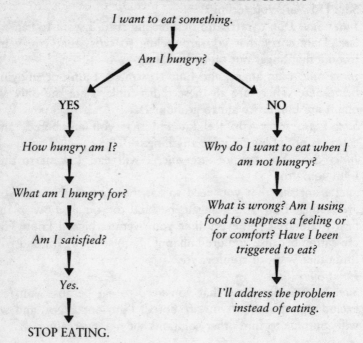

I want to eat something.

Am I hungry?

YES

How hungry am I?

What am I hungry for?

Am I satisfied?

Yes.

STOP EATING.

NO

Why do I want to eat when I am not hungry?

What is wrong? Am I using food to suppress a feeling or for comfort? Have I been triggered to eat?

I'll address the problem instead of eating.

If we use all our energy to keep our feelings in check, then we have very little left over to enjoy our lives, and we end up depressed and depleted. It is as if we have thrown a blanket over ourselves and we are living our lives covered over, and in the dark. Compulsive eaters use food not only to cover up their feelings but also to escape from them. In the instant that we are eating we change our mood and feel better, but as soon as we stop we feel bad again. Feeling fat creates a constant low-grade depression and we use eating to escape from this uncomfortable feeling, creating an endless vicious cycle.

That blanket over our feelings not only cuts us off from our own feelings and causes us to overeat, it also limits and restricts us in our relationships with others. Perhaps you can think of someone you know who is emotionally cut off. Think about how difficult it is to talk to them or to be close to them. In order to communicate with others, to experience real intimacy with other people, we need to be able to open up and share our real feelings with them. If you can't do that, you can't really be close to anyone.

Where do you fit in? Do you ever have difficulty knowing how you are really feeling? Do you have difficulty telling people what you really need, and how you are really feeling? If the answer is yes, the next chapter sets out to help you.

6

Stamp, Rage and Fret So That You Can Sing and Dance: Learning to Live with Your Emotions

'It is such a secret place, the land of tears.'

SAINT-EXUPÉRY

I remember very well that three days after my first husband died some neighbours came around to see me. I began to cry. The husband immediately said in a paternal tone, 'Now tut tut, pull yourself together.' I looked at him incredulously: 'My Stephen is dead and I must pull myself together?!' What I actually wanted to do was shriek and pull my hair out and run around frantically screaming about this nightmare I was in. I was never going to see Stephen alive again. Never. No crunch in the gravel of the driveway when he arrived home from work. Three days ago I was living with, sleeping with, planning to have another child with a gentle, loving man. Now

I felt as if everything was gone, and I had nothing, nothing.

Why should I have to pull myself together? I needed to scream for Stephen to please come home. In some cultures, when somebody dies, the bereaved wail and tear their clothes and shriek for days, and then they get on with their lives. Life does go on after somebody has died. If you have grieved, if you have allowed the pain and the anger and the outrage to rip through you, then you can go on and live a healthy life. If you don't grieve, but pull yourself together as our society encourages you to do, then part of you will stay frozen around the grief you are protecting, part of you will always be guarded, scared, worried that you might fall apart. Expressing your feelings is much healthier and saner.

Putting your hand in a flame will damage your skin, and pain is the alarm that makes you pull your hand away and prevent further damage. Our feelings can be the same important indicator system. They are a message from our bodies which tells us exactly how we are responding to what is going on around us. Our feelings help lead us away from unhealthy situations and towards healthy ones. If you feel anxious or angry in a situation, it is a warning to you to change that situation. If on the other hand you feel happy and contented, then you can leave things be. If you can become more aware of how your feelings are changing moment to moment, and day by day, then you will be sitting in the driver's seat of your life. If you are not in touch with your feelings, you are being dragged along helplessly behind the car.

Sharon came to see me because she had gained nine pounds in the three months since she had separated from her husband. We talked about her eating habits and she identified that she did most of her overeating at night. Now that she was living on her own she had stopped having a cooked meal at dinner-time and instead would have several snacks in front of the TV before going to bed. I asked her how she felt when she was at home alone watching television. 'Fine,' she said, and went on to talk about how the previous evening she had bought a packet of snowballs and every time she had gone into the kitchen she had eaten one. 'I was bored and lonely,' she said. 'I cannot believe I got through a whole packet of snowballs.'

Notice how, initially, when I asked Sharon about how she felt when she was home alone, she immediately answered that she felt fine. Then in the next breath she said how bored and lonely she was. She had said how she was feeling but she herself had not noticed what she had said.

Sharon thinks that if she stops eating snowballs at night then all her problems will be solved. The snowballs are not actually the problem, the boredom and the loneliness are. If Sharon does something about the real problem, if she hears her inner child's boredom and loneliness, restructures her evenings, sees her friends, meets new people, finds a new hobby that occupies her mind and her hands, then she won't need to eat snowballs at night any more.

George is a company lawyer, and his job is to act as troubleshooter when big problems flare up. He deals with hundreds of phone calls and crises every day. Sometimes the problems are small and easily solved, but at other times they can be massive and it is at those times that George has to use all his resources and energy.

As soon as the phones start to ring in the way they always do when a crisis is on, George starts on the supply of sweets in his drawer. I asked him why he does that, and in answer he shrugged his shoulders and said that he needs the extra fuel to help drive him through the problem.

I didn't agree, I think that he needs the food to calm himself down. As soon as the crisis hits George feels panic, he feels the pressure, his heart beats faster, he wonders if he can cope, so he eats, he knows no other way to cope with his feelings.

George has been doing the same job for fifteen years, and in that time he has coped with every difficult situation. What he cannot cope with are the feelings that come up with the situation. He automatically reaches for a doughnut to calm his nerves, a Milky Bar to stop his heart from racing, just as a smoker would reach for a cigarette, or an alcoholic for a drink.

There is another way: George can speak to his inner self. First he needs to acknowledge the feelings by naming them: 'I am really stressed out right now, I feel tension in my shoulders, I feel close to panic and I want to scream.' Then, if he needs to, he can act on his feelings. He could pace up and down, or punch a cushion. He could close his eyes and slowly count to twenty, he could learn deep breathing and relaxation. Then he will only open his food drawer when he is hungry. There are other ways besides eating to cope with our feelings – for Sharon, for George, for all of us.

I have a lovely seven-year-old son who has huge big blue eyes, with the longest pair of black eyelashes you have ever seen, an incredible sense of humour, and cerebral palsy. On Friday night I was having people to dinner and there was chaos. The phone kept on ringing, I was trying to get the dinner ready, and I glanced at Alan, my son, who was trying desperately to get a piece of toast into his mouth. I suddenly go like an octopus, one hand trying to steer Alan's hand in the right direction, the other hand stirring the soup, and then all six spare hands shoving any kind of food down my throat. Alan's leftovers, biscuits, garnishes from the meal. '*Stop! What is going on, Little Cherie? Where are you?*' 'I hurt, I hurt because I want my son to run and play, I want him to feed himself easily, I want him to be able to do things.' 'I know you hurt, sweetie, and I can understand why. Sometimes it's really hard but you can cry, you know.'

I cry and cry, the soup boils over. I cry some more, now I no longer feel like eating. I end up hugging Alan – I love him so much. My guests will have two courses instead of three, but I feel fine now. That night I write in my journal that I need to cry every time I feel sad about Alan not being able to walk and talk and do the things that other children find so easy. I remind myself that he has the best sense of humour of any child that I know, that he is warm and cuddly and full of energy. I write in big LETTERS: Alan is happy the way he is, the best I can do for him is to love him as he is.

A few months ago I got a call from a friend who lives in South Africa to say that he was in London for a visit. We made arrangements to meet and I put the phone down and headed down the stairs to the kitchen. I was not hungry, so I asked myself what I was feeling. 'I am *excited*, I am so *excited*!' Joy at the prospect of seeing him so soon barrelled through me. I remembered that when I was young and got excited my parents told me to calm down. 'You know what happens when you get excited, it will end in tears,' my mother used to say. The only way I knew how to calm myself down was to eat.

Once I realized what I was doing, I had the freedom to choose to do something different. So I continued my dash down the stairs and then turned right back up again, and then down and then up, shouting 'Hooray' as I went realizing that there is no one around to raise an eyebrow any more. And I didn't give food another thought.

If You Are Aware of Your Feelings, and Are Able to Express Them, You Will Stop Overeating!!

Most compulsive eaters eat to stuff down their feelings. Some people suppress their feelings by turning to things like drugs, alcohol, shopping, exercise, work and sex. We turn to food.

Initially as you stop using food to damp your feelings down you may feel really strange, as if you are losing control, but you are not. You are literally becoming a new person, a person with real feelings. Actually, by giving up food to control your anger, pain, anxiety and depression you are taking back control, real control over your life.

Day to day and month to year we go through a whole spectrum of feelings, feelings which range from joy to pain. Joyful feelings fill us with lightness, energy and a sense of well-being. Painful feelings can be dark and scary and sap our energy. We feel emotions in our bodies, they are what make us truly human. If we learn how to pay attention to all our feelings then we can get to know who we really are. But sometimes it is easier to say, 'I am fat because I ate twenty-six snowballs' than it is to say, 'I am lonely, I am afraid.'

If we name the feeling, if we say out loud 'I am lonely,' 'I am in pain,' then we can step beyond the loneliness. And the pain. There is a real person underneath all those layers of fat-blocked feelings, a person who once knew how to laugh, and sing, and dance and be angry and cry. A person who had energy, heard the birds singing, and got excited about dewdrops and rainbows. Someone who was truly awake.

In my work with dieters and compulsive eaters I have noticed that of all the emotions people experience there are a few that most of us have particular difficulty expressing. These feelings are pain, anger, and anxiety. I feel it is worth exploring them in a bit more detail to explain how exactly you can learn to express and deal with them.

Emotional Pain

Liz was forty-eight when I met her and she said she just could not stop eating. One night during a session on self-esteem, we were doing an exercise on what messages our parents might have given us about ourselves. Liz put her hand up to say that since we had begun the discussion about parents she had been feeling really 'emotional'. I asked her what she meant by emotional and she said she was feeling a burning feeling in her chest.

'When was the last time you cried, Liz?' I asked.

'Oh, last week I went to a movie and as it ended I had a few tears in my eyes.'

'Did you feel emotional then?'

'Yes, but not as strongly.'

'So, Liz, for you when you are in pain, when something is really hurting you, you feel emotional and you have a burning feeling in your chest?'

'Yes.'

'Would you like to tell us a bit more about what happened to you as a child?'

'Everybody used to say that my mother was weird, she used to rant and rave a lot, and the whole family revolved around her needs and her wants. She used to lock herself in her bedroom and scream and scream, usually about running away or killing herself. The first time I heard her threaten to kill herself I was so scared . . .'

By this stage Liz could barely talk because she had begun to sob out loud, a real cry from her heart. I handed her the box of tissues, and the group silently sat around her and let her cry out all her anguish. Her neighbour put a supporting hand on her back, and eventually the storm passed. Afterwards her face was soft and young. She said she felt like dancing, because she felt as if a ten-ton weight had been lifted from her shoulders.

Many people spend their whole lives running away from emotional pain. Whenever I begin a new workshop I know that for the first two or three sessions we are going to speak about weight, and eating, and getting slim. Then, after we all feel safe enough with each other to go one level deeper, we begin to talk about what the real problem is. That is when emotional pain surfaces. People talk about unhappy events in their childhood, about abortions that they had twenty years ago, about teenage broken hearts, about people they loved who have died, about divorce, they talk about loss, rejection, and pain.

If somebody does cry during a group session, then they are usually embarrassed, they apologize for 'breaking down', as if somehow by crying they have let themselves down. It takes me a while to reassure them that IT IS OK TO CRY. We have the ability to cry because it is the way we release our pain. Scientists have measured a brain chemical in tears which is not present when our eyes merely run, which shows that crying is an actual physical way of releasing emotional stress.

Holding on to our tears does not make our pain go away. Until we find some way of expressing the pain that has built up over the years it will stay inside us, weigh us down, slump our shoulders, and take our energy away. And so we eat.

We have learned to eat rather than to cry even though eating merely anaesthetizes the pain, it does not take it away. When we are in pain we can eat until we have gained five stone and then we can lose weight, and regain it, but the pain will still be there like a tumour, it eats at us, gnaws at us.

Some of my clients say to me that they fear if they start crying they will never stop. We are terrified of our pain, and we try and hide from it. The first time I really felt my pain, it was as if a dam had burst, it felt as if it would never end. I remember pulling my legs into my chest and sobbing, 'It's sore, it's sore,' and it really was. I cried for all the times I had been rejected, for the times I had been lonely, for the years I hated myself for being fat. But once I had confronted my pain the first time, I realized it would not kill me. Even though the pain ripped and roared through me, even though it left me bruised and battered for a while, feeling the pain ultimately brought relief. The bonus was that the more I cried, the less I overate. I will say that again, the more and more I cried, the less and less I ate. Now I always cry when I am sad, and that frees me up even more to eat only when I am hungry.

Now, if I feel pain building up, I usually arrange some time and space where I can be alone with my tape recorder and then I listen to special weepy songs, like 'Philadelphia' (Bruce Springsteen), 'Don't Give Up' (Peter Gabriel), and 'I Believe in You' (Neil Young). I use the emotional music to help start the tears so that I can have a good cry. After I am through, the sky looks somehow bluer, and the grass greener, and I feel the relief. Until the next time.

Maggie came to see me in a rage. A few months before, she had expressed a lot of pain around her relationship with her mother. She had felt much better after having done this and had thought that the pain would now be gone for ever. Unfortunately, she was wrong. Pain is part of living. Whoever decided that all fairytales should have a happy ending was wrong. Life is not like that. There will always be pain. There will also be joy. It is healthy, though, to be aware when you are in pain, to feel the pain, to cry and then go on; later, when you are sad again, to cry again.

I know that it is usually not appropriate to burst out crying in public, so if you find yourself in a situation where it is impossible to cry, you can just acknowledge the feeling inside you. Say to yourself, I am ready to burst into tears and I cannot because there are people around. Then give yourself a mental hug and treat yourself gently until you can get the emotional release that you need.

In my childhood, I don't remember when I stopped crying, but by the time I was fourteen and Arnold told me that he thought we should stop seeing each other, I had already learned to smile, even though I was hurting inside. Whenever anybody in my family cried my father would snap at us to stop immediately. He probably could not stand his own pain, and if we cried it would be harder for him to continue to shut his own pain out. Whenever my mother looks like she is about to cry, she forces herself to smile; she believes that you must push the pain away and keep very busy. No wonder I learned to stop crying when I felt sad or unhappy.

I wonder what patterns you learned from your parents about pain? What happened in your family when you cried? Did they allow you to cry, did they hold you when you cried? How did your mother behave when you cried? Your father? Did your mother ever cry in front of you? How did she react when she was upset? How did your father? Where in your body do you feel emotional pain, that is, how do you feel when you are about to burst into tears?

How do you respond to your pain, do you allow yourself to cry?

How do you suppress pain? Do you use food to do it?

It may help you to spend some time writing down the answers to these questions. With this new self-knowledge, you may well find the comfort of release which tears can bring.

Anger

Alice was five minutes late, and from the minute she joined the group I knew that she was feeling really uncomfortable. She spoke in short sharp sentences and she was restless in her chair. I asked her how she was feeling.

'I feel sick,' she said. 'I stopped at Safeway on the way home and bought piles of food and binged on it.'

I asked her how she was feeling before she went to the store, and when she still didn't know, I suggested that she describe her day.

'I got up this morning and instead of having time for breakfast, I had to clear the kitchen of the utter mess that had been left by my husband. Then I got to work, switched on my computer and realized that I had somehow deleted all the fucking work I did yesterday. I tried to explain to my boss what had happened and she dumped on me and told me that I would have to stay late today to finish the contract. Well, I did not stay late and I did not finish the contract and I do not care, and I still feel sick.'

'What feeling were you eating away when you crunched into the food that you bought, Alice?' I asked.

'Well, it's not fair, my boss wants me to be superhuman, and my husband expects me to keep the house even though I work as hard as he does,' she replied.

'Alice that's what you are thinking, but what are you feeling?' I asked again.

'Well, I am angry,' said Alice. 'But what's the use, it won't get me anywhere.'

Most of us in the group could see and hear that Alice was really very angry. The more she spoke about her day, the angrier she became. Her voice became tauter, her breathing tighter and her face was looking really strained. But she obviously found it difficult to identify and express her anger.

When Alice was young, anger was not allowed in her home. She was always told that anger was one of the seven deadly sins, and an angry lady is not a real lady. Now, when Alice was angry, she immediately ate.

Someone in the group suggested that Alice should put a cushion on the floor in front of her and pretend that it was her boss. (We often do this in the group.) At first Alice looked embarrassed, but then she allowed herself to erupt with anger. She started off by speaking loudly, and banged her fists down to emphasize her words. As she got deeper into her anger she began to hit the cushion harder and harder and she began to shout. Then suddenly she stopped. 'I feel like a real idiot,' she said. 'I feel like I am going to explode, like I am losing control, and I don't want to.'

'You don't look like you are losing control,' said another group member. 'I felt so relieved when you began to hit the cushion, after I noticed you talking with all this pent-up anger inside you.'

Alice was reassured, and started punching the cushion with renewed vigour. The next thing she said was, 'Whew, what a relief.' **THUD THUD**. 'I AM REALLY ENJOYING THIS NOW.' **SLAM BASH**. Alice's anger did cause an explosion, but not the one she feared: she had let the anger explode outwardly, harmlessly, away from herself and out of herself, away from others.

I often do an exercise in the group where I ask participants to draw a picture of their anger. I supply huge pieces of paper and lots of black and red crayons because these are the colours that everybody uses. As I walk around the room I usually see sparks flying as people draw volcanoes, tornadoes, rocks flying and explosions. Anger is an explosive emotion. Anger seethes and writhes and bubbles and steams, it needs an outlet, anger needs to be let out. If we keep the anger inside us it builds and builds like a pressure cooker with no valve on it. If we keep the lid on our anger and carry it all around inside us, just imagine what will eventually happen. All those volcanoes, all that steam inside us. Just as we learn to eat away our pain, so we learn to eat away our anger. Food becomes our pressure valve. We get angry and we just do not know what to do, all we know is that we feel awful, we feel as if we'll explode. We turn to food, we eat, we hate ourselves.

Anger is an important instinct. It is a defence that is there to protect you. I remember reading about a woman who had been dragged into the bushes in a park by a man whose intention was to rape her. As she realized what he was doing she felt a rage that she had never felt before and she screamed in a voice she had never used before. The man got such a fright that he ran away. Now I am not saying that you can always frighten off a would-be rapist with rage, but in this case this woman used her anger to protect herself.

Yes, but Cherie, I hear you ask, how can I express my anger without losing control? Without hurting someone, without living to regret it?

Expressing anger does not mean you need to lose control. Our emotions make us who we are. Our feelings are part of us, and anger is one of those feelings. We confuse anger with aggression, so anger frightens us, and many people believe that we should never get angry. Wrong. Anger does not have to hurt other people. It doesn't need to lead to any form of verbal or physical violence. Think how a child shows he is angry – he will stamp his feet, shout, cry out, slam the door. If you are angry, say it, let it out.

Does anybody you know regularly lose their temper? Losing your temper is a result of not managing your anger. Little bits of anger build and build until the pressure becomes too much and all the built-up anger explodes. I remember one night at home when we were all sitting around watching television. My mother was knitting and my father asked her to stop. She said no, as she enjoyed watching TV and knitting. Suddenly it was as if a volcano had erupted. My father got up and threw the tea-tray down on the floor, breaking cups and sending liquids flying. He had totally lost his temper. He did not lose his temper because of the knitting and the TV, but because of all the other little bits of anger that had been building up inside him during the day. It was a frightening incident in my childhood, and I became wary of my father after that, even though his anger had not been directed at me.

How Do You Respond to Your Anger?

You may find it useful to sit down and write down answers to these questions:
Where in your body do you feel anger? Do you usually allow yourself to express anger? Or do you suppress it by eating? Were you allowed to express anger as a child? What makes you angry?

Make a list of all the people you are angry with right now. Choose one of the people from your list and pretend that they are sitting opposite you. Tell them why you are angry with them, allow yourself to let go and scream and shout and beat a cushion up if you wish. Let the anger out. It is a wonderful release.

If you really give yourself permission to feel your anger, you can set yourself free from it. Here are some of the methods I use to express my anger, apart from beating up that poor cushion:

I let the anger fill me with energy, and I go and exercise furiously.

I go into a room where nobody can hear me, and I scream.

I stamp my feet and jump up and down.

I take my old hockey stick and beat a pile of carpets.

I play loud music.

I find something to clean, or scrub something vigorously and say I'm angry, angry as I do it.

Anxiety

I think that we would be really surprised if we could measure the amount of food that we consume to calm ourselves down. Anxiety is a huge trigger for non-hunger eating. Babies become very anxious when they are hungry, and they usually calm down when the first few gulps of food are swallowed. When we become adults we continue to use food as our adult dummy and tranquillizer.

I am anxious right now. This book is overdue, I need hours and hours more writing time. I need calm space and time. I don't have it, I have workshops in Glasgow every second night, and I am holding a workshop for forty people this weekend in London. There is no milk or bread in the house. My life is full to the brim with things I have to do, and places I have to go.

The anxiety is in my arms as a tremor. It is in my chest as an unpleasant pressure. My breathing is shallow and sharp, I am sweaty and trembly. I ate too much muesli at breakfast, I hardly tasted it. I had a scone with my tea, but I wasn't hungry. The food calmed me down for as long as I was eating it, but as soon as I stopped the anxiety came screaming back. As I write this, I realize I am at long last surrendering to the anxiety. I am acknowledging that it is there, giving the feeling a name. And immediately, it has begun to lose its charge. I begin to practise my breathing exercises, I breathe deeply into my stomach, I breathe out and pause before the next breath. In and out, in and out, calm air, calm breath, I tell myself that I do not have to be perfect. The anxiety dissipates. Thank goodness.

One of the biggest causes of anxiety is that we have such

rich imaginations, and we keep on imagining things going wrong. We are about to do something or go somewhere and we picture disaster in our minds.

I remember, on one such anxious occasion, I was driving to Edinburgh to begin my first workshop there and all I could think about was food. I started my usual dialogue with myself:

'Are you hungry?'

'No. Food, I want some now!'

'Well, why? What are you feeling?'

'I want some *food*.'

Eventually it came out. I was anxious, so anxious. I had started to imagine nobody would turn up for the talk. I worried that the people who did turn up would leave half-way through. The more I thought about it, the more anxious I felt.

When I became conscious of my anxiety, I decided to imagine a happy picture instead, I forced myself to imagine people clapping as my talk ended, I pictured the hall sold out. I began to feel much better, and by the time I arrived I was really calm.

As it happened, that talk was my one and only real disaster. Seventy people attended who all decided that they would carry on going to Scottish Slimmers, no matter what I said. It was as big a fiasco as I had imagined, but I felt a lot better having arrived at the talk without eating five chocolates to calm myself down.

There is also a big difference between healthy and unhealthy anxiety. If I am about to take an exam, or attend a very important business meeting, then a certain amount of anxiety is understandable, even beneficial. Healthy anxiety can give me the extra energy and motivation to apply myself to whatever is causing my anxiety. But I have come to see that most compulsive eaters suffer from unhealthy anxiety, which is energy-sapping and destructive. They worry, constantly. They immediately see the dark side of any situation: 'Oh, no, I'm going to a party and I'll be the only fat one . . . Oh, no, I have been given more responsibility at work. I'm sure it's going to be too difficult . . . Oh, no . . . Oh, no.'

The best way to deal with anxiety in the short term is to start a dialogue with your anxious, frightened inner child. Acknowledge her feeling, reassure her and tell her that you will handle things if they do go wrong. Just keep on speaking. Reassuring words, warm supportive words. You can of course also look at the situation that is causing your anxiety and see what can be done to prevent the same thing happening again in future.

For long-term anxiety and stress management you will really feel the benefit if you use short simple relaxation exercises like deep breathing and relaxation, as taught for example in ante-natal classes. These techniques are outlined in Dr Sandbek's book *The Deadly Diet* (see Book List, page 268), and they are also taught at yoga, meditation and relaxation classes.

Where are you now in your journey to overcome overeating? Well, you have successfully negotiated the first step, which was to discover the link between your feelings and your overeating. We have just finished examining the second step, which was all about learning to re-acquaint yourself with your suppressed emotions, learning to recognize them and express them. You are now ready to begin the third step: how to nourish yourself without using, or abusing, food.

7

Thunder Thighs and Fattism: Accepting Yourself

'I know these legs look as if they could kick-start a Boeing, but they are my legs, and they are fine. They walk when I want them to walk, they sit when I need them to sit. They are my legs, so they are fine.'

JENNY, A COURSE PARTICIPANT

When I started to follow the principles of conscious eating I found it really hard. I was not dieting, but I was still obsessed with my weight and I was still overeating. I still could only catch glimpses of a life beyond my weight problem. I felt I was stuck.

Then I had an experience which gave me a huge push in the right direction. I noticed that my friend Paul had changed enormously after he had attended a personal growth workshop. He seemed to like himself so much more. Paul tried to explain how the five days of the seminar had changed him, but he could not find the words. He said he felt as if he was riding a bicycle without stabilizers for the first time. He encouraged me to sign up for the seminar so that I could see for myself what had caused this big change in him. I trusted Paul, and I was eager to undergo the same experience as he had, so I impatiently waited for the end of the month when my five days were due to begin.

The first day we learned how most of us, from an early age, learn to protect ourselves from others. Instead of saying what we want to say and doing what we want to do, we start to put on an act, we create a person who we think will be acceptable to others. This is called our false self, and it is behind this false self that we hide our vulnerable true self. Often our act is so successful that we lose sight of our true self, and the false self takes over completely. Nina, our seminar leader, said that during the next five days she would invite us to get beyond this act, back to our true selves, and to rediscover who we really are.

The first exercise sounded really easy. All we had to do was stand up in front of the group, give our name, and state the reason why we had signed up to do the workshop. Nina asked for a volunteer to begin the process. There was an uncomfortable silence, so I rehearsed what I would say and stepped forward.

'My name is Cherie and I am doing this workshop for two reasons – firstly a close friend of mine found it very valuable, secondly I am planning to specialize in psychiatry and I want to learn why workshops like these change people so much.'

'That's interesting, Cherie,' said Nina. 'Now would you share with us the *real* reason why you are spending a lot of money and five days of your time at this workshop.'

'But I just told you,' I replied.

'I heard what you said, but I heard nothing of who you really are.'

Then the questions began. Nina skilfully asked me about my life and my relationships. She would not let me sit down.

For an hour I defended myself and my reasons for being there. The group agreed with Nina — everybody in the room could hear what I was really saying, except me. It took every one of those long, exposing sixty minutes for me to start hearing myself. When I finally realized why I was really there, tears rolled down my face.

'Would you like to begin again?' said Nina. 'Who are you and why are you here?'

'My name is Cherie and I am here because I am lonely and I need love.'

'Thank you. You may sit down.'

I was feeling really shaken, and when Nina told us what we had to prepare for the next day my heart sank even further. 'Tomorrow, I want you to wear under your clothes the sexiest, most revealing bathing suit that you own.' I spent a sleepless night worrying about the next day. Would we have to parade in our bathing suits like beauty contestants? I couldn't bear to expose my body. I only ever wore cover-up clothes. I would not be seen dead in anything the slightest bit revealing, never mind a bathing suit!

The next morning it was only the knowledge of how well Paul was feeling that made me squeeze into my swimsuit, and, with mounting trepidation, go along to the seminar. 'I am going to ask you to do something which for some will be easy and for others will be really difficult,' said Nina. My mouth went dry, and I could feel my heart pounding. The moment I had been dreading had arrived. 'I want each of you to stand up in front of the group, in your swimsuit, and say something about your body.' I broke out into a cold sweat, I could feel myself shaking, this was my worst nightmare. My swimsuit was black, and all I was aware of was how my rolls of pale white fat bulged out as the black lines of Lycra cut into me. Let me out of here, I can't do this. Mortified, I waited my turn, toying with various ideas like fainting, running away or just getting dressed and leaving.

Jenny went first. She had come dressed in fishnet stockings and a G-string. She stood up and I noticed that she had the biggest pair of legs I had ever seen. I marvelled that she dared let people see these fat legs. Then she said something that really shook me: 'I know these legs look as if they could kick-start a Boeing, but they are my legs, and they are fine. They walk when I want them to walk, they sit when I need them to sit. They are my legs, so they are fine.'

I did not listen to anything else for the rest of the day, and I don't remember what I said when my turn came along. I was bowled over by Jenny's words. Here was a person, a fat person, saying, 'Look at me, I am a woman, I have big legs and that is all right. I am not a bad person because I am fat, I do not need to hide my body because I am fat, I can walk and I can talk, I can make love and dance as well as any thin person. I am me. I am fine just as I am.' She did not feel compelled to apologize for her body, she did not talk about how much weight she was planning to lose, she simply accepted herself the way she was.

I was ashamed of my body. I hid my body at every opportunity. The only connection between me and my body was when I took a critical look at myself. I would get up every morning, look in the mirror and scream at myself about my weight. 'Look how fat you are, your stomach is disgusting.' By the time I had finished criticizing myself I felt so bad I would head for the kitchen and console myself with a bowl of cereal. Two bowls of cereal.

After this seminar, I worked really hard to try and find things that I liked about myself and my body, and focus on them. It was extremely difficult. Initially all I could think of was that I liked my eyes, so I decided only to look at myself from the nose upward. 'Good morning, Cherie, you have beautiful blue eyes.' Immediately I would feel better, and in general my morning overeating stopped. Gradually I started with the rest of my body, changing each insult to a compliment: those droopy boobs changed to a voluptuous bosom, that revolting fat stomach changed to cuddly tummy, and my thunder thighs changed to these strong walking legs.

I like my body. I am fine just the way I am.

In the first few hours of any workshop I always say that an important part of the journey to overcome compulsive overeating is that we need to begin loving and accepting ourselves exactly as we are now. There are always people who immediately react with horror at my suggestion. I remember so clearly as I write this how Nancy responded. She got up, pulled up her jumper, and grabbed hold of her rolls of stomach: 'You have got to be joking, like this fat, accept this fat!! I hate it, it's revolting!! What do you think I came here for? If I accepted myself as I am now then I wouldn't be paying to sit here, I would rather be at home watching television and eating chocolates.' Susan joined in: 'The only thing that stops me from curling up into a hole, and giving up completely, is my belief that one day I will be slim. If you are telling me I will be this weight for ever, well, I may as well shoot myself. Believing I will get thin is the only thing that keeps me going!'

'Hold on, you two,' I replied. 'If you accept yourselves as you are now, that does not mean you are accepting defeat, nor does it mean that you have to stay at the weight you are now. Imagine that you had a six-year-old daughter – when she got up each morning the first thing that you said to her was: 'You are so fat, just look at that stomach. You are revolting, if you did something about your weight you would at least be able to wear decent clothes. Well, you'd better wear black and cover yourself up, because your body is so revolting.

'If I spoke to a child like that I would know she is going to feel dreadful, she is going to want to crawl around in shame. And when she feels like that she will look for comfort, and the only comfort she knows is to eat something. That is probably how you criticize yourself each morning and that is probably why you need to comfort yourself with food. Imagine saying to the same child as she wakes up every morning something like: "Hello, sweetie, you look lovely this morning. How did you sleep and how are you feeling? I want to tell you that you are a really special person, and I love you." See the difference? She will feel loved, and if she does feel loved, she is more likely to do what you want her to, that is, not overeat. Her reward for not overeating will be weight loss, or at least weight maintenance, and that will make her feel even better about herself so she is less likely to need food for comfort. That child is your inner child.

'Look around at the different people in this room. I can guarantee you that the people who are size 26 and over wish they could look like the people that are size 18. Those who wear size 18 wish that they could look like the people who wear size 14, who want to look like the people who wear size 10, who of course would love to wear a size 8. No matter what weight you are you usually are going to want to weigh less. That is part of the syndrome of compulsive eating, we are as much hooked on getting thinner as we are on food. If you begin to accept yourself unconditionally now, this will lessen your obsession and also lessen your eating drive, otherwise the danger is that you will never be happy with yourself no matter how thin you are.

'Another reason to accept yourself as you are now is so that you will stop hating yourself because of the way you look. For years all that criticizing your body has done for you is send you back to the kitchen because you feel so bad. When you stop criticizing yourself, you will have much more energy available to go ahead and create the future that you really want for yourself. If criticism and self-loathing helped you lose weight, I would see only thin people in my groups.'

After years of nagging at yourself and lambasting your body it may seem strange and difficult to start giving yourself compliments. In Chapter 5 we spoke about how we all have a critical parent inside us, and that it is this critical parent who takes over when we yell at ourselves.

It is difficult to switch the critical parent voice off – after all, it has had free reign for many years. If you like you can try this exercise: think of the part of your body which you like the least. Start to criticize that part, really give yourself a blasting. Now notice who is talking – is there an image behind the voice? Does the voice remind you of either of your parents?

Be aware of the tone of voice your critical parent uses and also how often you speak to yourself with that voice each day.

Once you have identified the voice, you can begin to answer it back, tell it to shut up, and switch it off. Then replace the criticism with something kind, with praise; acknowledge yourself for doing your best.

When we have done that exercise in the group I usually follow it with a more lighthearted one. I tell everybody to divide up in pairs, and reveal to their partner which part of their body they are most embarrassed about. Then they are both told to point to the other's embarrassing body part in turn and laugh out loud. It may sound stupid, but it is cathartic. If you can stop being ashamed of your big bum, your loose tum and your waggly hips, you will get everything more into perspective.

When you overeat your critical parent will immediately kick in and say something like: 'I cannot believe you ate all that cheese, you are so fat and you are going to get fatter.' As you get to know that voice, you can answer it back in a sensible adult voice: 'I was hungry for cheese, I enjoyed it, and there is no way that one helping could make me fat. *And* I would prefer it if you did not call me fat please. I have a lovely curvy shape.'

Do try to learn a way to switch off that nagging voice. The minute you are aware that thoughts about weight, eating, and losing weight are beginning their familiar run through your head, try shouting STOP at yourself. I like to imagine that I am scrawling S T O P! in big black letters across a white screen in my mind, or that I am screeching to a halt in front of a big STOP sign in the road. Once you have stopped the destructive thought, you need to replace it with a constructive, kind thought. If you do not, the blank space that has been left will soon be filled with criticisms and accusations again. Replace the obsessive or critical thought with a new positive message, for example, I am a good friend, I have great taste, my hair is curly and shiny, I am fine the way I am.

Setpoint Weight

Perhaps at this point you may think this book is written by a confused person. First she spends pages and pages telling me how to eat, and stop overeating so that I could lose weight, then she says that it is actually fine to be overweight and that I should accept myself as I am.

To tell you the truth, initially, I *was* confused. When I first began setting up Weigh Ahead workshops, I asked an advertising agency to design a brochure for me. They came up with a glossy sheet which shouted in big black letters, 'Never diet again, lose weight by eating what you want.' And it had a big photo of me with a huge grin biting into a piece of cake. Later on, a course participant said to me, 'Cherie I am so pleased that I heard you talk before I read your brochure. It reads just like the advertisements from the diet industry, it seemed to promise weight loss as the ultimate goal.' I read it again and, with embarrassment, I had to admit that she was right. I made a decision to throw all the remaining brochures away. Perhaps, at this late stage in the book, I need to ask for your forgiveness for using the word 'slim' in the title. Unfortunately I do not know of any word in the English language which can describe the process of finding your natural weight. There is no neutral word that I can think of that describes the normal state of being in between 'thin' and 'fat'.

What my brochure should have said was: 'Stop dieting, stop being at war with your body, eat when you are hungry and allow your weight to settle at the level which nature intended.' 'But what level is that?' I hear you ask. And I'll say it again, the level which nature intended. At some point in our dieting lives we will have been presented with a 'goal weight'. A doctor or diet counsellor will have weighed us, measured us and then looked up what we should weigh according to the 'normal' weight–height tables.

But how do we know what normal is? How are these tables valid? Think of the infinite assortment of different noses, eyes and ears that people are born with. Who says what is 'normal'? We come in all sorts of different body shapes and sizes. Some of us are short, and some tall. Some of us have big hips, small waists, enormous breasts, or tiny feet. Imagine how boring it would be if we all looked exactly the same.

Since we all look so different, how have we been persuaded that all people of the same height should weigh the same? The goal weight tables that many doctors use have left a very important variable out of the equation. It is that each of us is born with our own unique setpoint weight.

Setpoint weight is a weight range that your body instinctively attempts to maintain. Just as the colour of your hair and eyes is programmed into your genes, so too is your weight. Instead of thinking about a specific goal weight, you can redefine what your natural weight is in terms of a setpoint weight range. I believe we are each born with a prescription for a certain weight range, and no matter how we diet and binge, left to itself our body will always attempt to return to that weight.

When Sally turned thirteen she was the tallest and biggest pupil in her year. She was 5 feet 8 inches tall, and she weighed thirteen stone. She went on her first diet when she was fourteen. She remembers the exact day. The school nurse had come around and she had been given a note to take home. The note was in a brown sealed envelope but Sally knew exactly what it contained: 'Dear Mrs Anderson, We have weighed your child today and she is well above the weight recommended for her height: she weighs 13 stone, but according to our tables, she should weigh 10½ stone. We advise that you put her on a diet, and a diet sheet is enclosed.'

Sally had been so embarrassed. The nurse had announced in front of the whole class that she was too fat, and had taken her along to the doctor. 'Fat as a sausage, young lady,' he said. 'If you don't lose weight, you will be a wallflower at all the parties, none of the boys will dance with you.'

Sally walked home with the letter, and a new image of herself. She kept on imagining the next school dance: Frank would ask her to dance, but he would run away as she stood up and he saw that her body had turned into a sausage.

Sally followed the diet the school doctor had given her, and lost weight, but then she regained all the weight she had lost, went on another diet, lost some more, and regained it and lost it again. I met Sally twenty years after her first diet, and she weighed sixteen stone. After a year of eating when she was hungry, stopping when she had had enough and exercising four times a week, Sally's weight dropped to fourteen stone. And stayed there. She came to see me again, as she felt that she would like to lose some more weight. I asked her to fill in a chart recording her weight fluctuations over the years. When she had done so it became obvious that Sally had in fact reached her setpoint weight.

The first clue was that her whole family had an 'ectomorphic build' – that is, most of the women in Sally's family are large. That already tells us that Sally's setpoint weight is likely to be high. The second clue to her setpoint weight was in the chart she filled in: every time Sally had been on a diet, she would lose weight until she weighed around thirteen stone, and then she would stop losing weight. When this happened she would try to reduce her calorie intake even more, but though she sometimes did manage to lose more weight on a starvation diet, she would become so ravenously hungry that inevitably she would begin to binge and regain the weight. Whenever Sally was between weight loss diets she would gain weight, and when her weight reached fourteen stone, she would stabilize at that weight. Four years before I first met her, however, Sally had become really depressed and had been compulsively eating and dieting her way up to sixteen stone.

Many people I know have gone to slimming clubs, lost weight to within five pounds, ten pounds or even a stone of their goal weight, and then, despite restricting their calories, have not been able to lose another ounce. It is frustrating to diet without the reward of weight loss, and a binge is almost inevitable. I believe that these people have come close to their setpoint weight. Sally's setpoint weight range is probably between thirteen and a half and fourteen and a half stone, the weight she was programmed to be when she was born. She is a tall shapely woman. If Sally had been left alone when she was thirteen perhaps she would have stayed in her setpoint weight range and would never have become a compulsive eater.

Sally has a choice. She could insist on weighing under her setpoint weight and aim to weigh eleven stone, but in order to do that she would have to starve herself on two lettuce leaves a day for the rest of her life. Or she could live comfortably within her setpoint weight range – which after taking some convincing is exactly what she has chosen to do. Sally exercises regularly, she eats what she wants when she is hungry, and her weight has stayed around fourteen stone. All the energy she used to spend alternately worrying about her weight and eating, she now has available to spend on her life. She has begun studying part-time for a law degree, and taken up hill walking and tap-dancing lessons.

Susan Kano, in her book *Never Diet Again*, proposes that underweight and overweight should be understood in terms of being above or below an individual's setpoint weight, not a general goal weight. A very thin person may look underweight but be just right for her physiological setpoint, and conversely someone may look overweight, but so too be found at her natural setpoint weight. It is no use fighting against this setpoint weight, it is inherited from your parents and your body will fight to stay at that weight. Chronic dieting, and the accompanying weight loss followed by weight gain, bumps up your setpoint weight, because when you diet your deprived body makes you hungry and your metabolism slows to a fat storage and conservation mode.

Because we are living in the era of idealized thinness, many people spend their whole lives battling to be under their setpoint weight, at a terrible cost. Several studies have been carried out to determine the effects of living under our setpoint weight, such as the Minnesota study, conducted by Professor Ancel Keys during the Second World War. To assess the effects of starvation on people during the war, he reproduced the effects of starvation in his laboratory. Thirty-six conscientious objectors, young healthy men, volunteered to live at the University of Minnesota for the duration of the experiment. The volunteers, who were of normal weight, were found to have 'high levels of ego strength, emotional stability, and good intellectual ability'. None of the men had any previous interest in their weight or in dieting, and they began the experiment in high spirits. Their normal food intake was reduced by half – this is quite usual by slimming diet standards.

The results of the study are remarkable and significant. As weight loss began the participants showed a variety of negative symptoms, including becoming increasingly irritable, preoccupied with food, apathetic and depressed. Many of the men found it impossible to stick to the diet, and when they did break the diet by secretly sneaking food, they felt guilty afterwards and made 'half-crazed confessions'. Their reduced energy and alertness, their apathy, decreased sexual interest and social isolation because of the diet, affected their lives dramatically. Some wanted to stay in the lab all the time because they were frightened they would not be able to stand the food temptations outside. Some of the men even began having long binges followed by self-induced vomiting. The effects of the semi-starvation diet lasted long after the experiment was over; subjects continued to experience cravings for certain foods, some became more self-conscious about their weight, and some put themselves on another diet afterwards. Many of the men also became obsessed with recipes and with cooking. These were people, remember, who, before the experiment began had *no particular interest* in food, and now some even said they wanted to become chefs!!

These men had begun to show all the early symptoms of compulsive eating after only three months on a diet: they became obsessed with food, they had begun to focus obsessively on their weight, they binged secretly and felt guilty, and they had an urge to overeat when the diet was over.

Similar experiments have also shown that when the participants in this type of experiment stop dieting, their hunger is insatiable. Many report eating huge meals and still feeling unsatisfied. In another study, also conducted in the USA, after a diet which had caused their weight to drop below its normal level, subjects reported eating up to *10,000 calories a day* and still feeling hungry.

When dieters drop their weight to below setpoint, their bodies cry out for food, need calories. They will crave high-calorie foods, wake up in the night hungry, irritable, depressed, hungry, hungry, hungry. The naturally slim volunteers who participated in these experiments went on a huge long binge after their diet was over, but they could argue that this was only normal under the circumstances. On the other hand, dieters who go on a binge after a diet tend to scream abuse at themselves, they think they are weak-willed, they blame themselves for having no self-control. The naturally slim volunteers understood that their urgent hunger was a reaction to their weight loss, and indulged their cravings for high-fat and sugary foods. When we diet to below our setpoint, we try and fill up on Diet Coke and carrots. But can you see – the ravenous hunger is your body's way of going back up to its setpoint. Our bodies will always strive to return to their setpoint weight because that is the level of optimum functioning in all aspects of life, physical as well as emotional.

So there is no fighting it? I hear you ask. The good news is that you *can* affect the level your weight settles at within your setpoint weight range. Regular aerobic exercise will help your body to defend the lower part of the range. Eating healthily will have the same effect: that means low-fat, low-sugar, low-refined foods, with plenty of fresh fruit and vegetables. Oops! Now that sounds a bit like a diet.

The difference is that if you exercise to 'burn calories'

and achieve a certain weight and hip measurement, you are stuck in the diet mentality. But if you discover the pleasure of regular exercise for fostering a sense of physical and mental well-being, a side-effect will be that this regular exercise will help you maintain a lower setpoint weight. Similarly, once you have stopped dieting and once you have satisfied yourself by eating all previously forbidden foods, if you choose to live healthily by eating a balanced diet, your body will maintain a lower setpoint weight. Eating healthily means making qualitative not quantitative change – eating well not eating less.

Judy had never felt the need to diet until her youngest child reached secondary school. It was about that time that she noticed that the shorts that she always packed for her summer holidays were really tight. Lately her husband had been ragging her about her rounded figure. She tried watching what she ate, but nothing changed, so she decided to join a slimming club. Lucky for her, she just could not tolerate the weighing and measuring and food restrictions so she gave up the diet. At the same time she read an article about how we all go up a size or two as we age. She had worn her mother's wedding dress at her own wedding, but only now did she remember that her mother had gone up two sizes over her lifetime. Judy is one of the lucky ones: she accepts her changing shape, and has no shame about tucking into macaroni cheese with the rest of her family. She has foresworn dieting once and for all.

Most of us will gradually gain weight as we age, except for some people with a small-boned, wiry build. Women who diet to try and fight against this natural process are more likely to suffer from osteoporosis, cardiac problems and earlier death than those who allow this natural middle age spread to happen.

My own weight has fluctuated a lot since I gave up dieting. After I had heard Jenny love her legs in her fishnet stockings, I decided that I was always going to be round, and my task was to learn to accept myself as I was. I did have a goal, though – my goal was to eat when I was hungry, and to work at understanding and changing the pressures that caused me to

eat when I was not hungry. That was three stones ago. My
weight has slowly but surely gone downward since then. But
it was not a steady downward path: my weight has fluctuated
up and down on the way. When I stopped dieting I gained ten
pounds, but over the next two years I lost forty pounds. As soon
as I stopped losing weight, I began to put on weight; I gained
ten pounds in the first six months and then another ten pounds
after Alan was born. Then I started to exercise regularly and I
steadily began to lose weight again, until my first husband died
and I could not eat for months; I lost so much weight my bones
stuck out. I could not sleep at night, I was cold all the time, I
worked compulsively, I was irritable. Then I gradually came to
terms with my loss, worked less, cried more and my appetite
finally returned. It was real ravenous body hunger. When I did
eat food it tasted heavenly. I would have a huge meal and still
be hungry for more food. This ravenous hunger stayed with me
until I had regained most of the stone and a half I had lost after
Stephen died. Because I had dropped below my setpoint weight,
my body was sending ravenous hunger signals until my weight
went back to its comfortable position. I never weigh myself now,
but over the past two years my clothes size has not changed. I
exercise regularly and I love fresh and wholesome food. But I
eat the occasional chocolate and pudding when I feel like it.
I am perfectly content for my weight to fluctuate. When it is
cold I eat more hot puddings, stews and thick soups, and when
the weather is warmer and I cycle and swim I always lose a few
inches.

When I speak about setpoint weight there are always one
or two people who begin to panic; they are worried about
what their setpoint might be. Actually I would ideally like you
to throw your scales away and forget about how much you
weigh altogether. But I know that you may be worrying about
your setpoint weight, so here are some guidelines to help you
estimate your setpoint weight range if you wish to.

If you began dieting when you were an adult then it is easier
to estimate what your setpoint weight range is. Your setpoint

weight will be close to your normal weight as an adult before you began dieting. If you began dieting as a child, before you reached your adult height, then it will be more difficult to estimate your setpoint weight, because that first diet would have interfered with it.

If you really want to estimate your setpoint weight range, it is useful to do a weight–time chart, that is, a graph of what has happened to your weight over the years. On the bottom axis of the graph plot out your age in years, and on the vertical axis fill in either your weight, or your clothes size. Fill in your weight or size fluctuations over the years as well as you can remember. Indicate in a contrasting colour the times when you were taking regular exercise – this will enable you to see how exercise affects at what point your weight settles.

What you will be looking for on the graph is an average weight, times when your weight was relatively stable, while you were not dieting. The weight that you tend to return to after dieting is likely to be close to your setpoint weight, although it may be a bit higher than your natural setpoint because of your body's metabolic rate change in response to dieting.

If you are eating when you are hungry, and stopping when you are satisfied, your weight will eventually settle at its optimum setpoint range. Programmed into our genes is a setpoint weight range of approximately one stone. That means that your weight will settle somewhere in that range or fluctuate within it according to what you are eating and how much exercise you are taking.

Candice is 5 feet 6 inches tall, and after years of dieting and compulsive eating she began this programme weighing fourteen and a half stone. After six months of eating only when she was hungry her weight had dropped to twelve and a half stone. She then began exercising by going to the gym three times a week, and six months later she had lost another six pounds. By now she had had her fill of the fatty and sugary foods she had been deprived of, and she began to choose healthier food. Her weight has now settled at eleven and a half stone. Her setpoint weight

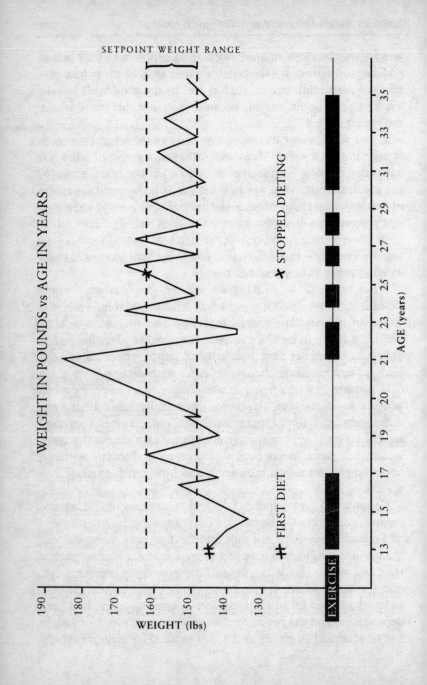

WEIGHT IN POUNDS vs AGE IN YEARS

SETPOINT WEIGHT RANGE

✗ STOPPED DIETING

⨱ FIRST DIET

WEIGHT (lbs)

190
180
170
160
150
140
130

AGE (years)

13   15   17   19   20   21   23   25   27   29   31   33   35

EXERCISE

range is between eleven and a half and twelve and a half stones.

Sam, on the other hand, is also 5 feet 6 inches, but had been on a rigorous diet and exercise programme, so she weighed just under nine stone when she first came to see me. She was cold all the time, irritable and weepy, couldn't sleep well because she was so hungry, and had stopped menstruating. After some counselling she realized her compulsive exercising was unhealthy, and she adapted her exercise programme to a more relaxed pace. She also allowed herself to eat when she was hungry, and gained a stone and a half. Once she was in her setpoint weight range all her symptoms disappeared.

It doesn't matter what you weigh, it matters that you are comfortable. Eat spontaneously when you are hungry and use your energy for being alive.

Prejudice

I was raised in South Africa. As a young child it seemed perfectly acceptable to me that black people went to separate schools, worked as servants, and used different hospitals, buses and trains from ours. It seemed normal.

When I was fourteen I came to Europe and for the first time I was exposed to a different point of view. I have a vivid memory of reading a magazine which contained an article about racial oppression in South Africa. Only then did I begin to see that what was happening in South Africa was wrong, brutally wrong. I lived in a system which indoctrinated me to accept that one sector of our society, merely because of the colour of their skin, should be subjected to inferior treatment.

There is another equally oppressive and blind prejudice alive in our society today, which everybody seems to accept without question. This prejudice is based on judging people by how slim or how fat they are. We see somebody for the first time and immediately classify them into one of two categories. Thin or fat.

In my groups, I sometimes ask what words people associate with a 'slim person', and with a 'fat person'. Often the words used to describe slim people include 'in control', 'happy', 'dynamic' and 'successful'. On the other hand fat people are 'sloppy', 'unhealthy', 'no will-power' and a 'failure'.

If you think about it, there are of course many slim people whose lives are a mess. There are also many extremely success-ful fat people. All of us, thin and fat, have different lifestyles, we all have different degrees of health, will-power, aspirations. Yet fat people routinely suffer rejection and abuse by society — a society that cruelly judges an overweight person as somehow second-rate.

I was shocked when the six-year-old son of a friend of mine told me about their recent holiday to the south of England to visit Uncle Davie and Aunt Joan. Part of the holiday news was obviously a well-rehearsed family piece, because six-year-old Graeme puffed out his cheeks, Dad stuck out his stomach, and both chorused in unison: 'Aunt Joan has got so fat, yuuuch!!'

Children are taught to be prejudiced against fat people from a very early age. They hear their parents make disparaging remarks against fat people, they watch when their mother looks in the mirror and she groans about an extra inch, and they hear her say that she does not want to get as fat as Mrs Smith next door. By the time children are of school-going age they have been taught about the demon fat. Fat is bad, children hear, fat is unacceptable, and they grow up as prejudiced as their parents are.

In America a study was done in which children were shown six drawings: a normal child, a fat child, a child in a wheelchair, a child on crutches with a leg brace, a child with a facial disfigurement and a child with a hand missing. The children were asked to put the pictures in order from the one they most liked to the one they least liked. With a very few exceptions the children liked the normal child most and *the fat child least*.

The medical profession doesn't help either. Many doctors

are extremely prejudiced against patients who are overweight, which is not justified by the medical evidence (see pages 45–48). Their prejudice affects the way they see and treat their overweight patients. Several of my clients have actually been told that their doctors would refuse to treat them unless they lost weight. I have been so angry when I hear how hurt people have been by some of the comments made by their doctors: 'If I were as fat as you I would shoot myself, rather than die the way you are going to die, from fat overload.' 'Well, what do you expect? If I was carrying five extra stone around, my knees and hips would also crack under the strain – first lose a stone and then I will prescribe the pain-killers.'

Liz said that she is scared to see her doctor, 'Because even when I broke my finger by catching it in a window, he managed to blame it on me being overweight. I went to him with chest pain and he said I should lose weight. Meanwhile it turned out the pain was referred from an ulcer, which has nothing to do with me being overweight, but of course he blamed it on my weight.'

Doctors who are fattist get their prejudice from society, not from medical evidence. Obese people are seen as undesirable patients and somehow it is acceptable to refuse treatment to such an individual. I am angered and outraged at such doctors, who dare to allow their prejudice to cloud their judgement and treatment of these patients.

The media, the movies and the models have done much to fuel this prejudice against fat people. An obvious example is how the media concentrated on the weight of Princess Diana and of Sarah, the Duchess of York, when they were both in the public eye. Diana is congratulated on her elegance and slim figure, never mind that she was reported to have suffered from bulimia. Sarah was always compared to Diana, and when she gained weight after her first pregnancy, the criticism was relentless. Many people sniggered as Sarah was renamed the Duchess of Pork. Of course she was redeemed when she lost weight again – 'from fat Fergie to svelte Sarah'.

The average size for women in the UK is size 16. A minority of *only 8 per cent of women are naturally a size 10*. Why then are all models, in fashion photographs and advertisements, women who are in the minority? I find it amazing how everybody blindly colludes to keep this prejudice going. We are continually exposed to images of people who are not representative, we see only models and actresses who are thin. Even companies promoting large sizes tend to use size 12 models – that's ridiculous, and insulting.

Imagine if every time you opened a magazine you saw models who were a variety of sizes. Pages of the magazine filled with real women: short women, tall women, fat women and thin women, all walking, talking, laughing, beautifully dressed. Wouldn't it be wonderful to see reality on the fashion pages, not clothes and designs which are only suitable for eight out of every hundred of us, but clothes which all of us could enjoy?

Most modelling agencies will only accept girls who are ultra-thin, and according to reports many of these models suffer eating disorders. The only way they can keep their weight down and stay within the body requirements for their job is to throw up every time they eat, or stop eating at all. In fact the incidence of eating disorders has risen dramatically.

It was not always like this. A very interesting study of *Playboy* centrefold models showed how the statistics of Miss America changed: between 1954 and 1978 she became one inch taller, and five pounds thinner. Normally from age thirty your weight goes up a little each year. The weight of fashion models has gone down every year.

This abnormal fashion trend is having a dangerous effect on women. We have become totally obsessed with trying to look like the Ms Perfect of the nineties. Every magazine we pick up has some article on how to change your body, lose weight, look better, exercise more, burn this away, cut out a rib or two, let the plastic surgeon suck out or cut away some fat, buy this make-up. We are so used to these messages that we accept them blindly and we are driven to obsess about changing our bodies.

Rubens and Renoir were artists who painted the beauties of their time: full-figured, round and lovely women. The voluptuousness of these women oozes out of the paintings. Real bodies, thighs and hips, and wonderful soft flesh − which would nowadays be called cellulite. I noticed the same thing in a poster shop the other day, when I looked through a collection of posters from the fifties and sixties. Marilyn Monroe, Jane Russell, Lana Turner − these women were our role models then. Marilyn Monroe was a size 16. Sexy meant curvaceous and well-covered. Now sexy means thin, too thin, impossibly long, elongated, insubstantial like a Barbie doll.

Recently I visited Fiji, where big women are considered to be the most desirable. I saw fat women walking around proudly, aware of their sexuality, aware of the effect they were creating. If I had seen them on a beach in the West, they would be covering up their glorious womanly bodies. They would hide away, spend their money on diet products, and they would be ashamed.

If we grew up in a culture which said that fat is perfectly acceptable, that fat people are sexy, then we would probably have masses of thin people desperate to gain weight, they would buy drinks called Fat-Fast, join clubs called Weight Builders . . .

Sally's eyes filled with tears as she told me how her life had been. She comes from a family who are all large, and she has been above sixteen stone for most of her life. She has really suffered because of this. 'People snigger at me at the bus stop; one day a group of boys called me a fat cow, and other people standing around laughed. I nearly died, I thought that when the next bus came along I would just throw myself under it. When I do get on the bus I squash myself next to the window and try and get as much of my thigh and butt up the side so I don't take up too much room. I get so embarrassed when I spill over on to the seat next to mine and squash the person next to me. And horrors when I have to get out at my stop when the bus is full. People actually groan out loud as I ask to push past them.

'I have a friend but she pretends to not know me when others are about, she says it would not do her image any good to be seen with a fat girl. I am so scared to go to places where I might have to squeeze through somewhere tight, or sit in a chair that is too small. I shop at Evans, that is the only place I can find clothes that will fit me. But I always take a Marks & Spencer bag with me to hide the Evans bag in. I get so ashamed when people see me there.'

We all suffer from fattism, slim or fat. When Meg said she wanted to lose weight, the whole group shouted at her, because to all of us she looked really slim. 'If you think I look slim, come to my office one day. The other women who work there are all size 10, and they let me know it. When I came into work the other day someone had left a magazine on my desk and it was opened at the page advertising Nutra Slim. They all make comments about me. One of them even suggested I start smoking to help me lose weight.'

Women vs. women: I was in the steam room in my gym in the company of two other women, who were in their early twenties. I wondered if they were ballet dancers because they were thin as reeds and every muscle on their bodies was sculpted by exercise. As they lay down on the wooden benches one leaned over and grasped three millimetres of skin on the other's stomach. 'You really have got a big stomach these days, you must do something about it,' she said. I gasped and watched as the one with the 'big stomach' wilted and said how she was not going to eat any fat for the next week. As I walked out of the steam room, I wondered what they thought of me. If one millimetre constitutes a big stomach mine must look gargantuan. What a way to throw verbal poisoned arrows at somebody, tell her she is fat.

Vicki was so happy when she went to the States and saw a store advertising jeans in extra-large sizes. She had been dying to wear jeans, but she was embarrassed to try them on in her local village. Now she was on holiday, nobody knew her and the store must really understand fat people because they are advertising for them, she reasoned. Vicki went into the store and headed for the racks of jeans. The sales assistant, the *thin* sales assistant, came up to help her, and Vicki shyly said she did not know what size she was as she had never bought jeans before. 'Oh, you will definitely be our biggest size,' the assistant said. Vicki let that one slide, but to her humiliation the biggest size did not fit. She handed the jeans back to the sales assistant, who said, 'Why don't you lose some weight and then come back, you really can't expect to get that backside into a pair of trousers.' Vicki swallowed back the tears and the huge lump in her throat – she had been so excited when she went into the shop, and now she was crushed, humiliated, crestfallen. She felt alone and heartbroken, and fat.

The prejudice against fat people causes endless amounts of pain, causes people to withdraw from life. The unwritten rules are that fat people should not dance, swim, or, heaven forbid, be seen without clothes.

I have nothing against thin people. If you are naturally thin and you eat spontaneously when you are hungry, then that is the way you are, and I encourage you to love the way you are. I am just totally outraged that because society has decided that only very thin is attractive all the rest have to suffer. I have good handfuls on my bum, and a nice rounded tummy. Short of taking a saw and cutting off some bone, my hips are never going to be size 10. I do not particularly want to look like a waif, I prefer to look like a woman.

I know I can be a lot thinner than I am now, but that would mean going against the natural trend of my body. I would have to exercise twice a day and live on a rigorous fat-free regime for the rest of my life. But what is the point? Will it make me a better person, a better mother, a better therapist? Will it make a difference if on my gravestone is written: Here lies Cherie, she was thin?

From a very early age we are given the message of how boys should be, and how girls should be. Boys can rough and tumble, be strong and change the light bulbs, girls on the other hand must be sweet and nice and *as attractive as possible*. From the minute we are born, we are sold the message of make-up and hair-do and to be alluring to the opposite sex.

The attention is all focused on what we look like, and not who we are. We will have grown up with a tendency to view ourselves as objects, to measure our self-value in terms of the way we look, not how clever, or successful, we are, nor how we relate to other people. What a calamity then if we are overweight. What a disaster if we start to grow old.

Our excess weight becomes an affliction – what a pity, such an attractive girl but she is fat – tut, tut. I grew up in a society prejudiced against me because of the way I looked. I was tried, judged and sentenced even before I had begun: you are a fat person, that means you are bad and unattractive, and you must spend your whole life trying to get thin.

We have a difficult task ahead of us; we need to change a prejudiced society. I believe we can. First we need to change it within ourselves and then we can work on other people. When we see an overweight person, we should comment on how soft and lovely they look. When we hear a 'fattist' comment, let's not be afraid to make a comment back about the objectionable prejudice being expressed. If someone jokes about another person's weight, we'll tell them we don't think it is funny – would they think it was funny if we joked about their bald spot, or the size of their nose?

We can all make a difference, to sway public opinion back to normal, so that tolerance will spread and we can all learn to live comfortably with the body we were given. In America the pressure group NAAFA (National Association to Advance Fat Acceptance), founded in 1969, is hard at work to reduce 'fattism'. It backs people who have been discriminated against because of their size and weight. The media are, to say the least, not very supportive of these efforts to get equal rights for fat people, because to them fat people are an obvious joke. Bryan Appleyard writes in the *Independent*: 'Soon they'll be waddling – sorry, sorry, marching – down Pennsylvania Avenue and President Hillary will be launching positive discrimination programmes . . .' And in their November 1994 issue, *Options* magazine asks: 'Fat rights – a big issue or a bad joke?'

The Americans are also way ahead of Great Britain in monitoring the diet industry. The FDA has put severe restrictions on slimming pills and amphetamines and the whole diet industry is currently under scrutiny. In 1992 the British government produced a paper, 'The Health of the Nation', which aims for a reduction in premature deaths from heart disease by reducing the prevalence of obesity. There is *no* mention of the harmful effects of dieting.

There are some moves in this country though. In 1992 Dietbreakers established a National No-Diet Day, and in the same year Labour MP Alice Mahon tabled a motion in the House of Commons which calls for legislation to curb the diet industry. The British Code of Advertising Practice has six pages of rules about slimming clubs, slimming products and what is permissible advertising copy for these.

In my talks I always tell the story of Jenny and her legs which could kick-start a Boeing, so through me she has touched many people. We need to stop hiding our bodies, to discard shame and step out and show ourselves whatever weight we are. If anybody says or thinks anything negative, that is their choice and their problem.

Recently in Western society there has been a great trend against discrimination against anybody because of their religion, race, sex, sexual preference or age – but we still have dispensation to discriminate against fat people. We realize that a person cannot help being the colour, age or sex that they are, but this tolerance does not spread to fat people. The overall consensus is that fat people are to blame for their largeness. Because it is their fault that they are fat, it is OK to abuse them.

My experience in group therapy has shown me that if somebody has a really strong reaction to what somebody else has done or said in a group, that person has something going on inside himself that needs attention. If somebody has the need to be super-nasty, he usually has a need or an inadequacy inside himself that clamours to be expressed. The person who makes a nasty fattist comment at a bus stop has a problem within himself. He may really dislike himself, or he may suffer from a terror of becoming fat himself, and that is why he is hitting out at others.

After all, your body is not an ornament for everybody to look at, your body is an instrument – your legs are for walking, sitting and standing, your heart beats, your diaphragm contracts and expands as you breathe. It is a wonderful instrument. Learn to enjoy living in your body. It is the only one you have.

If I tell five people about setpoint weight, and fat prejudice, and they each tell five people who tell a further five people, we can spread the word. But the most important people to tell are ourselves. Like Jenny who stood up in her fishnet stockings, be proud of your body, and tell yourself you are fine the way you are.

8

Learning to Love Your Body

'*I have never felt grateful, like many big women, for the mere attention of a man. I have never felt that I only deserved the leftovers that thin women reject.*'

DAWN FRENCH

'*Too fat to cross my legs, too fat to run,
too fat to say body, too fat to say fat.*'

IRENE O'GARDEN

When we become obsessed with changing our bodies, we become obsessed with food, and when we are obsessed with food we overeat. This chapter is about the fifth step, rediscovering your body: learning how to be at peace with your body.

As newborn babies we are totally in touch with our bodies. When we are hungry, tired, cold or in pain we become extremely uncomfortable and we cry until our needs are met. For some babies their needs are met a lot of the time, but for others things begin to go wrong from a very early age. We have two generations of people walking around whose parents ignored their hunger cries in favour of the clock. We were put down to sleep when we were not tired. We were boiling hot but were left with our jackets on. We were subjected to a denial of our bodies' needs. Sometimes our needs *were* met – we were hungry and Mummy came immediately and fed us and we experienced utter bliss and contentment; we were wet and cold and Mummy changed us, wrapped us in a warm blanket, and we felt wonderful.

From a very early age we started to look to the outside to try and make us feel better inside. When a baby is hungry for food and gets fed it feels total contentment. When a baby needs love and gets fed it learns to try to answer an inner need by eating something. That is the huge con about eating when we are not hungry. We are bored, lonely or tired, and we answer that need by eating something. The food perhaps helps for a few minutes but then we feel worse. We continue to search outside to try to make ourselves feel better inside. We are tired, so we have a coffee. We need a hug, so we eat chocolate. We learn to turn all our needs into a hunger for food. So we stay needy.

If we can move from looking to the outside to make us feel better and focus on how we are feeling inside, we will lessen our overeating. In order to answer our inner needs we have to be in touch with our bodies. A wonderful way of getting in touch with your body is to move, to exercise.

In my workshops I ask the participants to complete the following: 'If I woke up tomorrow and I was my ideal weight what I would do is . . .' I noticed that people filled in the same thing time and time again: 'I would exercise,' 'I would swim,' 'I would go to a keep-fit class.'

Karen is a good example. She is twenty-eight, 5 feet 5 inches tall, and weighs thirteen stone. 'My life would be so different,' she said, 'if I became thin. It would also be a lot less embarrassing; after I have walked up the hill to my bus stop in the morning I usually arrive huffing and puffing like a steam engine.'

'I think you could walk up the hill without puffing and panting, Karen,' I replied.

'No way, I am much too fat, just think, I am lugging three stone of weight with me as I go.'

'Yes, I agree, the extra weight is heavy to carry up the hill, *but* if you were fit you could walk up the hill without being short of breath.'

'You mean it has nothing to do with my being fat, but rather I just am not fit enough!!'

'That's exactly what I mean. You can become fit no matter what weight you are. There are many slim people who puff and pant, and who are not fit. Compulsive eaters tend to blame everything on their extra weight and when they say things like, "I can't walk, swim, hill climb because I am too fat," they are wrong. They cannot do these things because they are not fit, and you can become fit whatever weight you are.'

If I could give you one precious gift, one that was beautifully wrapped with ribbons and bows, I would give you physical fitness. It is the most wonderful feeling in the world to have your body toned up and able to move easily. By becoming fit I do not mean that you should be able to run a marathon. I mean that you can walk up a flight of stairs without panting, that you can take the garbage out, do the shopping, without becoming short of breath. I mean that you can live your life freely and not be encumbered by a body that is not being used to its full potential.

I know I am not alone in recommending exercise – you have probably heard it again and again. I am not telling you to run on the spot for half an hour, I am not telling you how to do enough sit-ups to get a flat stomach. But I need to include a section on exercise because I really want to convince you to make exercise as natural a part of your life as breathing is. Overcoming any eating problem is a hundred times easier if exercise is part of your weekly routine. If you already exercise, sit back and relax through this chapter, but if you are one of the people who thinks that two minutes of exercise is too much, then this chapter is for you.

When I studied anatomy in my second year at medical school I was totally amazed at the wonderful complex network of muscle, bone, vessels and nerves that our bodies consist of. Our body is an incredible creation, and it is built to move. Our legs are made for walking, climbing, running, our arms are for pulling, holding, swinging. We have the capability to walk for hours and hours every day. It is so natural to walk, to run, yet we sit in our cars or on the bus. We park as close to the store as we can get.

Have you ever asked yourself why you have so little energy, why you move with such reluctance, why you resist exercise of any description? I'll tell you why. First, remember how dieting decreases your metabolic rate? When there is a sharp decrease in the amount of calories that we ingest, the body reacts by conserving as much energy as possible. The less we move, the more energy we conserve. When your metabolic rate is decreased, you are going to be *ssssllllowwwed* down. You will have a resistance to using up energy. You will want to sit down, to send people to fetch you things, and you will be permanently tired.

This is a physical resistance to exercise, but for many, there is a psychological resistance to exercise too.

Angie was listening to her two friends talk about the aerobics class that they attended twice a week. It sounded like such fun. Angie longed to go with them, but when they had invited her she had immediately refused. She had said that she was busy on those nights, but that was not the real reason. Angie absolutely knew that there was no way she would appear in public in a leotard and tights, a size 18 leotard and tights. 'Can you imagine,' she thought to herself, 'me clumping around like a baby elephant. Never in a million years!!' Angie had been to watch the aerobics class once, and even though everybody looked as though they were really enjoying themselves, she noticed that everybody was thin, super-thin, size 8 in Lycra. *And* the room they were exercising in was surrounded by mirrors. Angie would not go swimming for the same reason – when she thought of herself in a swimsuit, she saw herself as a hippo among all the flamingoes. Poor Angie. What a lot of fun she was missing. If only she could be persuaded that what people thought when they looked at her was irrelevant, that she had a *right* to do things that she enjoyed no matter what size leotard she wore.

Ruth told me a story about her holiday: 'Everybody was sitting around the pool when a tall, confident-looking woman in a black swimsuit walked out on to the pool deck. She tested the water with her foot and then went up on to the diving-board, and with a wonderful, graceful dive she entered the pool. She swam a few lengths, energetically, then lifted herself out of the pool and walked the whole length of the pool and stood chatting to someone before lying down. It took me a while to realize that she was really fat, at least twice my size, but she was so confident, and walked so proudly, that she looked fine. I realized that I, on the other hand, usually wrap the towel around myself, creep towards the pool when I think nobody is looking, and jump into the water as quickly as possible. After I saw this woman I was emboldened, I got up and walked slowly to the pool without covering up in my towel, tested the water, and slowly got in. My heart was beating, and I felt deliciously naughty. Of course nobody even noticed me, but I felt different. I enjoyed it.'

Walk tall, stand tall, feel fine, no matter how wide you are. Usually the only person really bothered by how you look in a swimsuit is you. You are what you tell yourself you are, and you are perfectly entitled to walk, exercise or swim no matter how you look. Remember, if anybody is bothered, or makes comments about your weight, that is their problem. They'll forget about you in two seconds, it is how you feel about yourself that matters.

When I was at school, as I got more and more overweight each year the compulsory school cross-country race became more and more agonizing. I remember feeling hot and fat and so uncomfortable. I hated it. I also began to dislike the gym period, because I always seemed to be the only one who could not do the routines. Exercise became a real chore. Like a typical dieter I would either force myself to exercise as part of a diet, or I would not take any exercise at all if I could help it. I always felt big, ungainly, and movement was really difficult for me.

Years later, when I moved to Scotland, I was invited to an aerobics class which one of my neighbours ran from her home. There were only eight or nine of us in the class and we were all beginners. There were no fancy mirrors and nobody wore Lycra. There was just music, movement and we all had a lot of fun. This was one of the first times I had really enjoyed exercising, and a whole new world opened up for me. I suddenly realized that it was fun to move my body, no matter what weight I was. I had discovered a freer, lighter self within my body.

As I emphasize the need for exercise, please realize that this is *not* exercise to burn off the fat, as you have always been told to do by the diet books – the amount of calories that we burn up while exercising is laughable. However, I have already shown that regular exercise does have an effect on your weight in that it encourages your weight to defend a lower setpoint level. Also exercise can do much to help defuse some of the anxiety, tension and boredom that cause us to overeat. Exercise has lots of other benefits: for example, it increases the beneficial effects of cholesterol, and reduces the harmful ones. Did you know that regular exercise can improve your circulation and reduce blood pressure as effectively as medication? That it can help keep premenstrual tension at bay? That it can reduce the risk of diabetes? Or that people who exercise are 100 per cent more likely to find ways to relax and 300 per cent more likely to be able to relax when under stress? Exercise helps you feel good in mind and body. It means you need less sleep and have more energy. Exercise even works as a natural anti-depressant; it is a proven way to lift your spirits and improve your mood. And people who stay physically active into old age are much less likely to suffer from osteoporosis. Exercise keeps you supple and more mobile, and can prevent much of the bone loss which accompanies ageing.

Most of us wake up in the morning and immediately begin to think. We think about all the things we need to do that day, about how much weight we need to lose, we worry and think and worry. The more we think, the less aware we are of how we feel inside. It is as if we have cut ourselves off from the neck downward. The only attention that we give our body is when we look in the mirror and call ourselves fat. We need to learn how to feel, and we can only feel if we are aware of our body. Exercise is a wonderful way of getting in touch. When I am swimming I feel the water around me, over my legs, under my arms, I feel my legs thrashing the water as I kick. When I am at my step-aerobics class and I really begin to work hard I feel drops of sweat, my body getting hotter, my heart beating, my muscles warming up. Sometimes I feel as if I could fly. When I used to slump around the whole day all I had was my thoughts; now that I am fit I know I have a body, and since I am more aware of my body I can identify tiredness, stress, tension. I can also identify hurt, loneliness, all my feelings. When I am in touch with my body I am also in touch with my feelings; I don't need to eat so much.

Have you ever noticed how after you have been ill in bed for a day or two, when you get up you feel really weak and shaky and lacking in energy? This is because your muscles have begun to waste. The muscles begin to lose their energy store very quickly. Luckily this is reversible, and as soon as you use your muscles again they will rebuild. But the more you rest, the weaker the muscles get, the more resistant you feel to exercise. A vicious cycle builds up. The heart is no different from your other muscles in this respect; it needs to exercise to remain strong. In order to keep the heart muscle strong you need to exercise for twenty minutes three times a week.

Watch out though. The move from compulsive eating to compulsive exercising can happen so quickly you might not even notice it. Sometimes, after a stressful, tiring day, exercise can relax and revitalize me. But if I am utterly exhausted or ill, and I force myself to exercise, I am no longer listening to my body. When I plan my exercising around my food intake – I must have a workout because I hate a huge meal last night – I am not listening to my body. Missing an exercise class when you are tired will not cause you to gain twenty pounds overnight, and if you catch yourself on that destructive thought treadmill, stop. Listen to your body, eat when you are hungry, rest when you are tired, and exercise for fun, for fitness, *not* as a whip to make yourself slimmer.

How to Begin

I hope I have convinced you that exercise is fun and can make you feel better about yourself. If it has been a long time since you exercised, you must start off very slowly. Five minutes' more exercise today than you did yesterday is significant. You can even begin by just adding more energy to your daily life. Walk rather than take the car. If you have the car, park a few blocks away from where you are going. Do the housework with energy and vigour, do a few bum squeezes and arm lifts while watching TV, swing your arms as you walk. Use every opportunity to move your body, and whatever you are doing, do it with just a little extra energy.

If you are *very* overweight, and out of condition, stationary cycling on an exercise bike and swimming are the safest ways to begin building up your strength. This is not the place to give you a rundown on all the types of exercise available, but there are lots of different activities to try; whether you join a gym, start walking, go swimming, try dancing or aerobics, learn to play tennis or rock climbing, one type is bound to suit you.

Just remember exercise will free your spirit as well as your body – try it and see.

Sexuality

When I first planned this book, I had a lot of difficulty deciding where to include a section on sexuality. Shall I put it in the chapter on emotions, I asked myself, or in a chapter of its own? Then it became clear to me that it should go into the chapter about being in harmony with your body. After all, sexuality is an integral part of our expression of ourselves.

When we grow through puberty and adolescence our bodies change. I read somewhere about a girl whose parents took her out to dinner and gave her a beautiful gold chain when she got her first period – to celebrate her becoming a woman. I was so touched by this story. It was so different from the stories I hear most often, about being teased about budding breasts, about fathers who stopped playing with their daughters exactly at the time their hips and breasts developed. Stories about being sexually abused, by brothers, by uncles. Stories about being told to use separate wash-cloths because 'it' was dirty, being told not to touch ourselves 'down there'. Stories about building up fat on our bodies to be safe; stories about using fat on our bodies to say no.

When Elspeth saw the movie *To Sir with Love*, with her parents, she was puzzled by the scene in which Sydney Poitier, who plays a teacher, is really angry to discover something left by one of the girls in the classroom. Elspeth asked her father what it was that the teacher had found and she was really surprised when her father replied, 'Some disgusting female object,' in a tone that implied that she should not question him any further. Elspeth wondered what it was about herself that could be so disgusting. Her father also told her that he did not watch his children being born because he would feel strange about being associated with her mother after seeing all the 'yucky bits around the birth'. Elspeth concluded, after hearing all this, that the bits about her groin were actually quite dirty and disgusting, so when she started getting her periods at fourteen she was scrupulous about keeping clean. She also began to gain weight rapidly about then. During a particularly heavy period, she decided to wash herself directly under the bathroom tap. She was so surprised at the wonderful tingly sensation – until then she had not even known that her clitoris existed. As well as the messages about being 'dirty', Elspeth was always told never to touch – 'No hands in your pants please.'

Karri told me that she had sex with her boyfriend when she was fourteen. 'We were in his bedroom and he asked me to take my clothes off. When he put his penis inside me I lay there and let him, it didn't occur to me to say no, because he was so insistent. Even today when I'm with my husband if he wants to kiss we kiss, if he wants me on my stomach, I lie on my stomach, I lie there and watch and wait until he has had his orgasm.'

There are many variations on the stories told by Elspeth and Karri, but they all tell how many of us are brought up with a progressively increasing sense of estrangement from our bodies and our sexuality. We do not feel connected to our bodies, we feel as if our body is an object that is there to be clothed and looked at. We take this sense of alienation into our sexual relationships, and instead of joining in and asking for what we need we watch ourselves being touched, and worry about how fat we are.

At my evening sessions, I often read out the visualization from *Fat is a Feminist Issue* by Susie Orbach. I ask everyone to sit comfortably and close their eyes, and to imagine themselves at a party. First you notice how you relate to the people at the party, then you notice how this changes as you imagine yourself getting fatter and fatter. Then you imagine yourself becoming thinner and thinner and how you relate to others after that. After everyone has opened their eyes again, I ask each member of the circle in turn about their experience at this imaginary party. The results are often the same. Generally most of the women see themselves as flirtatious and sexy when they are thin, but when they are large they withdraw from the people at the party, and feel like hiding in the corner. *Some feel really relieved* at being able to do so. They feel as if being slim and sexy is too much of a burden, that if you are slim you have to be flirtatious and extroverted, that you will constantly have to fend off the unwanted advances of taxi-drivers and colleagues at work. So on a conscious level they want desperately to be thin, but unconsciously they need to stay fat.

Many of the women who feel this way are the ones whose adolescent bodies got them into trouble. They learned fast that their curves, their breasts, their mini-skirts brought unwanted leers and advances. So they got fat, and use that fat to give a message to the world: I am keeping myself hidden away in here and I am keeping you out.

Linda told me that when she was sixteen she went on the grapefruit and liver diet and lost two stone. She bought a tight mini-skirt and high-heeled pumps and proudly went off to town with her friends. Within half an hour she was terrified, she wanted to go home, because she was not used to the leers, the whistles, the suggestive comments. None of this had ever happened before. She borrowed her friend's jacket so she could hide her body away, and soon gained back all the weight she had lost. Somehow she felt much more comfortable. More stories about using fat on our bodies to protect ourselves, to deny our sexuality.

We don't need to say no by wearing a fat body – we can say no by saying no. No to kisses we do not want, no to anything that hurts or is uncomfortable. No to our partners if they want sex and we are not in the mood. Remember that if they choose to feel angry or rejected, that is their problem. There is nothing wrong with you or your sexuality. It is not a personal rejection of your partner, it is simply you honouring your needs and your body, and putting them first.

A long study conducted in Chicago found that women's sex lives are damaged more by being too thin than too fat. As the calories are restricted so does our appetite for sex dwindle. The results of the study showed that plumper women desire sex more often than thinner women. The more concerned the women were with their bodies the less interested they were in dating and sex. Kim Chernin eloquently expands this point in her book *Womansize*: 'A woman obsessed with losing her weight is also caught up in a terrible struggle against her sensual nature. She is trying to change and transform her body, she is attempting to govern, control, limit and sometimes destroy her appetite. But her body and her hunger are, like sexual appetite, the expression of what is natural in herself . . .'

The library desk on which I am writing has a message: 'I screwed a fat woman last night. She was fantastic, soft and comfortable.' Somebody has replied to this graffiti: 'She was probably really grateful to you – fat women hardly ever get laid.' We all know that this view exists; some people are not attracted to overweight partners, but there are also many men who enjoy and choose voluptuous curves and handfuls of adequate bosom rather than flat-chested, or over-exercised and unnaturally thin women. There is a dating agency in the UK for fat people who are tired of being rejected because of their size. Interestingly enough, well over half the men on their books are slim, and they want to meet large women.

Just as I encouraged you to discover the joy of movement in exercise, so too do I encourage you to rediscover the sexual being that you are, no matter what weight you are. Three cheers for role models like Dawn French, she is sexy and saying so.

As you begin to give more attention to your body, your real hunger for food, and your feelings, you can start to pay attention to your sexual needs and wants too. It will be a lot easier to let go sexually if you feel comfortable in your body, whatever weight you are. If you start calling yourself fat when you are having sex, your enjoyment temperature will plunge to freezing. If your fear of being naked with the lights on is stopping you, then you must face your vulnerability, and take the risk just the same. If you stop thinking fat, you will stop feeling fat. Rather, concentrate on delicious feelings. Revive your sex life with your partner and stay open and honest about your sexual relationship. Enjoy your sensuality, learn how and where you like to be touched, go at your own pace, it's all right to take as well as give.

Having an orgasm is not the major aim of making love, because everything that goes before and during and after is just as important. But pent-up sexual energy can lead to a lot of overeating and the way to release sexual energy is by having an orgasm. In fact one of the ways you can learn to nourish yourself without food is to spend an evening with your body. Low lights, music, body oil, fantasy and touch. Indulge in feeling good, and help yourself reconnect with your body.

Denise shared with the group how when she was a teenager she used to dream about Saturday nights with her boyfriend. She longed for him to hold her, and she giggled when she remembered how he would 'accidentally' touch her breasts. 'Now I dream about food just like that,' she says. 'I can go into orgasmic ecstasy about a good meal. I dream about food, I long for food just like I used to long for sex.'

For women to have changed the shape of their bodies as they have over the last three decades, they have had to eat less, much less. There was a change from home-maker, to wonderful body-maker. Sex was no longer forbidden fruit, but food was. Being fat has become more scandalous than being promiscuous.

The advertising agencies know this about women now. Some food adverts are blatantly sexual. Think of the message of a beautiful woman getting into a bath naked, and caressing a phallic-looking chocolate bar with her tongue and lips, or the

Häagen Dazs advertising campaign which mixes the visual metaphors of sex and ice-cream.

Food is food, and sex is sex. We only need to eat when we are hungry.

9

Nourishing Your Soul

'And she, who has such a great appetite for life, leaves my office one day, having talked with much passion and despair about her hatred of her body; and when she hugs me goodbye she turns aside. "I didn't want to press my stomach against you," she says.'

KIM CHERNIN

Carol, who came on my course, had a full-time job as a social worker, three children to ferry about, a home to run, a husband to cosset, and an ageing mother to worry about. She said that coming to my course was the first thing she had done for herself for years, beside eat. When she felt stressed and put-upon by the demands of her family and her work, she would eat something. It was the only way she felt able to fill the void that was left behind when she had given everything she had to give and it still was never enough.

In today's society it has become perfectly acceptable to give ourselves out every day, the whole day. We cook and clean and taxi and entertain. We are mothers, wives, working people, daughters and all-round caretakers. Compulsive eaters are often compulsive givers. We need to feel needed. We take care of everyone's needs except our own.

Carol shared her fantasy with the group: it was that she needed to have a major operation so that she would have to spend a few weeks in hospital. In her fantasy she would be in a nice clean bed and she would be looked after by attentive nurses. The pain would be a small price to pay: she wouldn't have to lift a finger, as all her meals would be served, somebody would clean her room, change her bed, bring her endless cups of tea, and her husband would have to cope with everything at home. What a sad fantasy. Carol desperately needed some pampering. She had absolutely no idea of how to do that for herself – even her dreams were not about tropical beaches and health spas, and the only way she could even *imagine* relaxing and being looked after was to be ill.

The more we give out without receiving anything in return, the more desperately hungry we get. We are hungry for care and attention, starving for love and acceptance, but the only way we know how to take care of ourselves is to eat something. We eat and eat and as we get fatter externally we continue to starve internally.

All this can change when we start to lavish some attention on ourselves. We need to learn how to nourish ourselves emotionally without food. We need to go back to school. We need lessons in how to be good parents to ourselves.

Often we have been raised to think that it is selfish to look after ourselves. Strangely, it works just the other way around. The more we take care of ourselves the more energy we will have available to take care of the people who need us.

Michelle was the third of four children. Her mother worked

full-time in a clothes store, and her father was often at home only on weekends as he travelled about for his job. When Michelle came home from school she would get her own tea and do her homework alone. When her mother came home from work, Michelle would be eager to talk to her and tell her about what was going on at school, but somehow her elder brother and sister always got in first. Michelle always felt inferior, as if she was much less important than her elder siblings. She carried this feeling with her right through school and nursing college. It was while she was training as a nurse that she began to diet; she was never successful at keeping her weight off and as she trod the destructive diet cycle she became fatter and fatter. Now not only did she feel not good enough as a person, she also felt fat. As the years went by she confused both those feelings into one – and her conclusion was, 'I am a bad person because I am fat.'

She did very well at nursing. In her assessments her superiors always remarked on how wonderful, caring, and giving Michelle was – she was able to anticipate and take care of everybody's needs, patients and staff. Michelle always read her assessments with a sense of surprise; she wondered who was this wonderful caring person about whom everybody was talking.

After she had lost weight on a diet, Michelle met and married Jim, and she continued her pattern of tirelessly taking care of everybody else, right through her marriage and three pregnancies. She went back to work after each baby was born, as soon as her maternity leave ended. She worked, baked, cleaned, mothered, and made lovely meals for her family every evening. She made them delicious creamy hot foods and puddings, while she ate cold low-fat food and lettuce leaves. She got the whole family involved in her dieting, so when she did reach out for something delicious, everybody, her youngest child included, would shout, 'Mum you are not allowed that!'

When I first met Michelle it took enormous amounts of convincing to persuade her to make some steps to take care of herself. Initially the only reason she would consider it at all was because she was so exhausted; she felt as if all her energy had been drained out of her, and she felt she couldn't go on. She felt so bad about herself, her self-esteem was at rock-bottom. She began by practising self-esteem building exercises, by looking at herself in the mirror every morning and telling herself, I deserve time and attention, I am fine as I am, I am a lovely person to know. I am valuable. Then she began to give time and attention to eating what she really wanted, when she was hungry. The next steps were really difficult for Michelle because she needed to learn to say no and take some time for herself. She decided to stop working into her lunch hour, and instead to use the hour to walk, window-shop, or just put her feet up. She also made some changes at home – the children each had to help with the housework, and she confronted her husband about how little he was doing in the home. In almost direct proportion Michelle ate less when she was doing more for herself.

So many of us just accept our role as caretakers to everybody but ourselves. We cannot be endlessly giving of ourselves, we must get something back. If you do not take care of yourself you will suffer the consequences – a loss of your health, of your self-esteem. You will continue to want to use food for comfort. Food, when you are not hungry, is not nourishment. A hug, a massage, an intimate chat with a friend, a walk in the park is nourishment. Dieting is a punishment, bingeing is a punishment; eating when you are hungry, and eating the delicious foods you are hungry for, is nourishment. If we nourish ourselves we will blossom, and have energy, if we deprive ourselves we will wither. And the choice is ours.

Perhaps it would help to imagine you are in a park with a group of children all running around and playing. You suddenly notice that one of the little children does not join in. She is too busy sweeping up the leaves, picking up after all the other children, and looking after those that are hurt or unhappy. You know intuitively that this little child is lonely, tired, and sad. What will you do? Your choice is to leave her, or to step in and help her. Perhaps the state that you are in inside is like that little girl. To help yourself, begin slowly by carving some time from each day that is exclusively yours, and build it up to at least an hour each day. At the weekend, negotiate some time for yourself, preferably a whole afternoon. This is your time, a time set aside so that you can take care of yourself. Pursue a new interest, take up an activity you loved doing when you were younger, but let go because there simply wasn't time.

I spend a lot of time talking this through with my groups, because it is so important. We have to replace our overeating with other nourishment, otherwise we will continue to use food. I always ask participants in a group to volunteer what for them constitutes something luxurious and pampering without eating – so that we can all trade good ideas on how to nourish ourselves. Whatever you decide to do, make sure, that it is just for *you*. And doing something once will not be enough – do try to arrange to pamper yourself regularly.

Here are some of the varied ways in which the members of one such group could think of giving themselves a treat:

'I'd phone a friend, a friend that I can really talk to, and tell her how I am feeling.'

'I'd give myself a pampering, a bath and a beauty treatment: manicure my nails, soak my feet, give myself a face pack, and then, if it is cold, wrap myself in a warm blanket, or comforter, with a hot water bottle, or in front of a fire.'

'Even if I only have ten minutes I can do some stretching exercises, or relax, or play with my cat.'

'I'd read one chapter of my book, or daydream.'

'I'd buy myself a newspaper or magazine, and read it cover to cover.'

'I'd like to write a poem, or try to write a poem.'

'I'd write in my journal – my Weigh Ahead journal!'

'Listen to my favourite piece of music.'

'Meditate, or go for a walk outside.'

'I try to visualize where I'd like to be in a year's time.'

'Paint or draw in vibrant colours.'

'Plan my next holiday.'

'I've learned to say no. No to taking on commitments when

I am already exhausted, no to spending time with people I don't
like, no to my soup being served cold in a restaurant, no to my
mother-in-law coming to stay. No.'

'Go to the cinema on my own in the afternoon.'

'Make love, with or without my partner!'

'If I have the time, and money, I go for a massage, a
facial, or just a swim and a sauna.'

'I'm saving up to go to a health farm, not a diet farm,
a place to relax and have all those lovely treatments!'

'Go shopping and spend some money on myself.'

'I'd ask my husband to give me a foot rub.'

'I'm learning to speak up for myself – when I want something
I ask for it.'

Susan went home after one such group discussion and asked
her husband to tuck her into bed and read to her – she told us
later that she loved it. May hired a cleaner, Adie arranged a night
out with her friends once a week. Kim took out a subscription to
a magazine – when it arrives she goes into the study, puts on the
answering machine and locks the door.

It was a few weeks after we had finished making the list of
non-food nourishers that Kim brought the topic up again: 'It's
lovely to take care of myself a bit more and give myself treats,
but I need much more than the occasional massage. Goodness
what will I talk about, think about, wish for and hope for if I
leave my eating problems totally behind? It seems strange to
say, but I am actually scared of being without it.'

Important question. Compulsive eaters use food and their
weight problem to fill a void, an emptiness which has been
inside them for a long, long time. In health we reach for warmth,
love, intimacy and spirituality; in this disease of compulsive
eating we reach for food. Food is an unnatural companion and
a poor substitute for what we really need. That is why we need
to really work at filling the gap that is left when we leave our
compulsive eating behind.

Like Sandy, who took leave of absence from her job, packed
her bags and went on a four-month trek to the Himalayas. Like

John, who started tap-dancing lessons, like Marie who began a degree in languages as a mature student, and like Larry who learnt to swim – as a sixty-third birthday present to himself.

As part of her journey to recover from compulsive eating, Margot decided to go to a meditation class which she saw advertised at her local Buddhist centre. The class was good and kindled an interest in Buddhism which she then explored and began to practise. 'I cannot believe the calmness and serenity it has brought me,' she said. 'What a difference from the chaos and confusion of my bingeing days. I'll never go back to overeating now, why would I when my life is so full and rich, with other things?'

Sandy had been raised a Catholic but had not been inside a church, apart from weddings, christenings and funerals, for years. 'When I was a child I was dragged along to church, and hated it,' she said. 'I eventually dropped the whole idea of religion in my teenage years because I tried to understand what God was, and couldn't. My compulsive eating was ruining my life. I knew I needed help and so I decided to ask God to help me. I only realize now that I do not need to understand what God is, my spirituality is personal and a *feeling*. A feeling within me. Now my journey to recover from compulsive eating has become a spiritual one. I am discovering a new relationship between me and God and my world.'

Despite numerous attempts, Shelley had not been able to fall pregnant. Instead of four extra slices of toast one morning she phoned a social worker to find out how she and her husband could go about adopting a child. It took several years, but when Shelley went to pick up her baby the longing that she had been eating away was, at long last, stilled.

Recovering from compulsive eating is an adventure: it means expanding our horizons, our lives and our relationships. The most important person to have a good relationship with, though, is our *self*. The final step of our journey is all about improving that primary relationship.

10

Food Is a Four-letter Word
. . . So Is Love

*'The wounded inner child is the major cause of addiction
and addictive behaviour.'*

My father always wanted a son. He often told us that in the
Far East people would bow in reverence to a father of sons;
our family, he said, would be sniggered at there. It became a
standard family joke that when my grandmother heard about
my birth, she told my parents to throw me out the window
because I was the fourth daughter. All very funny. Hilarious.

From as far back as I can remember I always felt there
was something wrong with me. That somehow I was different,
that I never belonged. I really tried hard to win my father's
approval though. *If I change, Daddy, then will you love me?*

In the beginning I tried to do boyish things, I played with cars instead of dolls, I accompanied him to all the rugby and cricket matches. That didn't work. Then I noticed that he was really happy when I got good marks at school, so I made sure that I always had an average well over 90 per cent. Many a Saturday night I spent with my school books when my friends were out having fun.

My high school leaving ceremony was one of the unhappiest nights of my life. I won every prize that was available to me. *If I win all the prizes, Daddy, then will you love me?* Each time I went back up on to the podium I felt more and more unhappy. Most bilingual, best actress, first prize, Head Girl. It was as if each thing that I had achieved made me feel heavier and heavier inside. Each award was a slap in the face, because my father continued to treat me in the exact same way he had always done.

On the surface nothing had changed, but inside of me something finally broke that night. Years of pain, years of the impossible frustration of being rejected over and over again, culminated on that night. Now, I can see how my father set me up for failure, how my mother was never there for me. Then, all I felt was despair. I finally gave up the struggle. I agreed that there was something very, very wrong with me. *I won't try and change any more, Daddy, I am not worth loving.* When everybody had gone to bed that night I went into the kitchen and ate a packet of biscuits, three bowls of cereal and two bananas. I was so full, I hurt.

The next day when I got up I just continued where I had left off and ate and ate. I hated myself for eating and I felt ashamed of all the weight I was putting on. I had no other way of dealing with the pain of being alive and feeling unwanted. I was deeply wounded, but the only place I could go to for love, for a dressing on my open raging wounds, was to food. The hole inside me could never be filled by food, but food was all I knew, so I continued to eat and I got fat again, but this time I got really fat.

Our parents, or the people who bring us up, teach us to be, teach us those crucial first pieces of knowledge. We learn their definition of what love is and their definition of right and wrong. We are exposed to their religion, their ideas and their friends. They actually mould us. We fill our minds with the information that they give us, and then we live our whole lives according to that information.

If we are born to a Christian family we are told about Jesus, if we are born to a Jewish family we are told that the Messiah is still coming. My father told me that fairies lived at the bottom of our garden – I believed him. My mother told me that when you are looking for a parking space you must tap the steering wheel and say 'Zelda, find me a parking.' When I am desperate for a space, I still do that.

While we are growing, we have a need to identify ourselves, to learn the answer to the fundamental question: 'Who am I?'

Our parents answer that question by providing a mirror, the reflection of ourselves that we see when they look at us. A normal, healthy mother reflects back to her child that he is acceptable, that he is loved. If a mother hates herself, a child will see that reflected and conclude that he is hateful. If a parent is nervous and fearful his child will feel nervous and fearful. If your mother didn't want to have you, you may feel as if you don't exist.

I was enduring a long wait at the doctor's surgery, in the company of a five-year-old boy and his mother. In the hour that we were there the mother looked up from her magazine only four or five times, and every single communication she had with him was a criticism. 'Stop that, you are a bad boy, be quiet, bad boy. Bad boy, bad boy.' All the time he was learning from her. When he asks the question, who am I? his answer will be what his mother taught him. I am a bad boy.

The Emptiness

Children who are growing need so much more than food, clothes, and a roof over their heads. They need to be hugged, they need to be loved. They need unconditional love and acceptance. We look to our parents to affirm the essence of who we are. We need our parents to love us exactly as we are. We plead for that love over and over again. Please love me, Mummy, don't look at me like that, Daddy, please say I am all right as I am. Please.

But unconditional love is hard to give, it clashes with a parent's instinct to teach her child to behave, to be in control, to do better. Most children are raised with criticism, they are constantly told to be quiet, to do better at school, to be good. Even normal loving parents do this, they say, 'Not now,' when their child clamours for attention. 'I'll play with you later.' Everyone suffers some rejection as a child. So imagine what happens to a child who is subjected to physical, sexual or mental abuse, or to children who are neglected or abandoned.

We keep our arms stretched out for as long as possible but eventually we decide that we are not worth loving, and we drop our arms and stop asking. At that moment it is as if our heart breaks, and then we live forever with a wound, a yearning, a longing. This wound, this 'hole in the soul' as John Bradshaw calls it, stays with the child as he or she grows into adulthood. People develop their own way of filling that hole – with work, with alcohol, with drugs, with possessions. Compulsive eaters use food to fill that hole, because eating will lift that sadness for the moment that we are eating.

What About Me – I Had a Lovely Childhood?

I was talking about the pain, loss and rejection we suffer as

children at a Weigh Ahead workshop when Annette broke in:
'But I had a lovely childhood, Cherie, my parents were sweet and
loving and kind.' 'So were mine,' said Josie, another workshop
participant. 'In fact I feel a bit of a fraud being here. When
all these other people start talking about being beaten up and
abused and abandoned, I feel like there is absolutely no reason
whatsoever for my eating problem. My parents were so good
to me. I was loved and cherished and given everything.'

In reply I told them a story I heard at a lecture given by
Jack Black of Mindstore. Richard and Susan were about to
be married and Richard was watching his future mother-in-
law prepare a roast. She rubbed the joint in oil, seasoned it,
and then before she put it in a roasting pan, she cut a slice
off and threw it away. 'Why did you do that?' said Richard.
'Oh, I always do that, it's force of habit,' said Susan's mother.
After they were married a few months Richard was watching
Susan prepare a roast, and he grinned as she rubbed it in oil,
seasoned it, cut a slice off and threw it away. A few months
later, Richard was helping Susan's grandmother prepare dinner.
He rubbed the roast in oil, seasoned it, and as he was about
to cut a slice off Susan's granny stopped him: 'Why are you
doing that?' she asked. 'I was pre-empting you,' he replied.
'This is something all the women in your family do.' Susan's
granny smiled. 'I had a favourite roasting pan and the cut of
meat I bought always needed a bit sliced off before it would
fit. I threw it away years ago, so no, Richard, you needn't cut
a slice of meat off the roast.'

Our parents had parents, and their parents had parents.
From generation to generation we learned so many things
that we have never thought to question. Even if your parents were good and loving people, there were probably times
when some hurt that they suffered in their childhood surfaced
and made them turn away from you or yell at you. Even if
our parents had the best intentions in the world, they themselves carried a wounded inner child inside – if you think
about it, you were often raised by an angry four-year-old,

hidden away in the five and a half feet which was your mother.

If either of your parents was a compulsive eater or an alcoholic or addicted to anything then it is likely that you will come out damaged. If your mother was obsessive about her eating and continuously worrying about her weight, how could she have been there for you, or taught you to be sane around food? If Dad was addicted to work and Mum felt abandoned by all the late nights in the office, who was there for you? Your dad may have said that he was working so hard to earn money to give you a better life, but if he wasn't there, for whatever reason, you will have felt abandoned as a child. Abandonment is life-threatening and painful to a child. If your mother was kind but had a low self-esteem, in all likelihood she will have passed that on to you. If you never saw your mother cry then you will have learned not to cry. Perhaps your parents were overprotective; that may have made you fearful. Any family traumas like unemployment, divorce, illness, death, will have had an effect on you. You don't need to blame your parents, it wasn't necessarily their fault. It doesn't mean you have to reject the happy memories, but it is important to face the hurt and pain as well.

Even if your parents had terrible things to cope with them-selves – if they were orphans, prisoners of war, or suffered terrible poverty, they had no right to abuse you in any way, and you need to say that to yourself over and over again. Don't insist that you had a happy childhood because you can't face the pain of admitting to the unhappy times.

If you are a compulsive eater, if your self-esteem is wrapped up in how thin or fat you are, then you can only benefit by looking at your childhood history. Not to point fingers at your parents, but rather to identify what you learned from them and to question whether you are still cutting pieces of meat off a joint for a pan that was thrown away years ago. Our parents had parents and our grandparents had parents. The pattern of parenting is usually passed down from generation to generation. Daughters of alcoholic fathers marry men who turn out to be alcoholics. Families which have rules like 'Do not talk about things' and 'Do not feel your real feelings' pass this rule through the generations.

I was having lunch with a friend, and she was sharing with me just how badly she had been treated by her father. I suggested that she see a therapist to work through her pain and anger, and she answered: 'I could never do that – I could never put my father through all that pain.' She was talking about a man who had physically and emotionally abused her and the rest of the family for years; and she didn't want to put him through any pain. Perhaps the truth is that she did not want to put herself through the pain of confronting him. In fact confrontation may not be a necessary part of facing up to the pain of your childhood. You could actually go through the whole grieving process without saying *one word* to your parents. The grief is inside ourselves, we need to hear ourselves say we were badly treated, we need to feel the pain and the anger, we need to tell *ourselves*, we need to confront ourselves.

Inner Child – Are You Serious?

Sometimes during a workshop when I begin to discuss the inner child, I feel the atmosphere change. After all, this is supposed to be a workshop about eating too much, so why all the 'psychobabble' about having an inner child? But by the end of the workshop, the scepticism has usually evaporated. By doing the exercises people have actually experienced their own inner child and they are thrilled by the experience.

The concept of the inner child is now widely used in therapeutic circles. There are a lot of books available on this subject. I love John Bradshaw's books. In my worst moments of the past few years his books became my friends; as I read them, I felt that at least one person understood. The following discussion draws heavily from his books, and if you are interested in a much more detailed description, see the Book List on page 266. I strongly recommend them.

Our natural inner child is who we really are deep inside – the part of us that is thrilled by something beautiful, who laughs out loud, who gets shy, who likes to be naughty, who falls in love and who cries at the end of a sad movie. If when you were a child your parents were over-protective, absent, if you were physically or sexually abused, abandoned, or brutalized with words; if your parents belittled you, made fun of you or tried to have an adult relationship with you; if they neglected you or did not allow you to express your feelings; if they were alcoholic, or work addicts, or compulsive eaters, your inner child will have been wounded. The child who was wounded has no way to cope with her hurt, pain and anger, so she kept it bottled up inside her. Outwardly she may seem normal but inside she is hurting, vulnerable and frightened. As we grow into adults so we carry our natural inner child with us, and we also carry the wound. *We grow into adulthood with this wounded child inside us*.

Several times during this book I have posed the question: 'Why do we, as logical thinking adults, do crazy things around food?' The answer is that it is your wounded inner child. She is the part of you that overeats. She is the one who will eat even though her stomach is bursting. She is the one who wants food all the time. If you have ever stormed out of a room, lost your temper, sulked, insisted that you are right when you know you are wrong, if you have found yourself behaving like an irrational five-year-old, then you are experiencing the behaviour of your wounded inner child – and, of course, when you have found yourself cramming your mouth with food you didn't even want.

Rubberbanding

Six months after I met my husband, Philip, we went on an eight-day cycling holiday in France. We cycled in the hot sun through the day, and then settled happy and exhausted each evening to enjoy French cuisine and red wine. I cherished every moment of those eight days. For the first time in five years I had been constantly in the company of somebody I loved and who loved me.

On the day we returned, our plan was to leave our luggage at Philip's flat; he would go to work and I would continue writing this book. All was going according to plan, until Philip got ready to go to work. I began to feel edgy, I kept on making excuses to delay his inevitable departure. I got angry, I said he should have arranged to take the afternoon off, I walked with him right up to the front door and I wanted to hang on to his sleeve. By the time he did leave I was sobbing. I felt as if he would never come back.

When I was four we moved house. Up until then we lived across the road from my parents' clothes store. In the new house they left for work early in the morning and returned just before my bedtime. I was left with a nanny, who sent me to my room to play on my own for most of the day. The house seemed big and dark and lonely, and the shadows that danced on the walls seemed evil and dangerous. I started to feel panic each time my parents left in the morning, I would hang on to their sleeves, I would walk with them to the front door. When they left I felt as if they would never come back.

The afternoon we returned from our holiday, Philip was not in the company of a thirty-four-year-old adult; the feelings that had been brought up had reminded me of my four-year-old self. As if a rubberband had been stretched between that feeling of abandonment while I was four years old and the feeling of abandonment when I was thirty-four. This is what is called 'rubberbanding', the connection made in your subconscious between things that happened in the past and things that are happening now.

The hurt and anger from years ago stays stuck inside us, and if something in our adult life reminds us of that hurt and anger we are catapulted back to that time and back to that feeling. Whenever you find yourself 'over-reacting' to a situation, when the feelings are too disproportionately intense for what has just happened, then it is a fair guess that your wounded inner child is remembering something that happened to her so long ago. The more stressful the situation is, the greater the rubberband. Now that you have started to talk to your inner child, you can start to identify those occasions when the rubberband takes over, and get to understand yourself better.

Relationships

Our wounded inner child not only infects our life by defiant eating, and by rubberbanding, but also by interfering in our intimate relationships. The first man you ever have a relationship with is your father, and your mother is the first woman. When Mummy or Daddy says 'I love you', we believe that the feeling that is there between the two of us is love. When we look for a partner we often choose a relationship which reminds us of the love we did or did not receive from our parents.

I have a client who is going through the break-up of her second marriage. Both times she married men who were alcoholics. Her father was an alcoholic, and he made the whole family's life a misery. My client keeps on trying to love men who are alcoholics. She thinks she wants to help them, but what her wounded inner child is really trying to do is *help her father*, stop her father from drinking.

Audrey lives with her husband, Tony. Audrey will not let Tony out of her sight unless it is absolutely necessary. She follows him around the house, questions him when he leaves,

begs him not to go anywhere. She even gets upset when he closes
the bathroom door. Audrey's mother left when she was two. Her
father worked, and Audrey was left alone or with childminders.
Before she married Tony she kept on falling in love with men
who were unavailable – either physically unavailable because
they were married or lived far away, or emotionally unavailable.
By watching Tony all the time, Audrey's wounded inner child is
making them both miserable, and unless Audrey deals with her
original wound she will make her worst fear happen by making
life so uncomfortable for Tony that he will leave her.

Chronic Depression and Low Self-Esteem

The 'hole in the soul' that is created when our inner child gets
wounded can cause a chronic, low-grade apathy or depression
which can drag around with us our whole lives. This yearning
for love and feelings of low self-esteem get confused in the
mind of a compulsive eater – we call this constant feeling
of unhappiness 'feeling fat'. And it is natural that we would
want to escape from this feeling. Notice how you feel as you
see the credits on the screen at the end of a good movie. It is
like coming back from another place. For the movie's duration
we have been totally transported to another world. We forgot
about our own lives, our own problems. It is only as the movie
ends that we come back to reality and thoughts of our lives
come flooding back. Eating and obsessing about our weight
problem is the same as going to a movie of our own creation,
because in that moment of eating, or thinking about how much
we weigh, we have effectively escaped from what we are feeling.
Food becomes our feel-good drug.

When we begin to untangle our past, uncover when and
why we became wounded, only then can we address the real
cause of our chronic sadness. If we gently expose our wounds
and then heal them, if we reparent our wounded inner child,

bring her out into a new loving relationship, support her and accept her, then we will not need to eat when we are not hungry.

11

Grieving and Growing

'As long as you eat compulsively, your life is about what
you eat, how much you eat, how much you weigh, and what
you will look like, be like when you stop eating compulsively.
Your pain seems to be about food, willpower, and looking a
certain way. But your pain is not about what it seems to be
about. And if you don't know what your pain is about, you
can't release yourself from it.'   GENEEN ROTH

In the last chapter, I showed how once we have become obsessed
with food we use eating as a method to fill the wounds left from
our childhood. When we stop overeating, we are faced with the
fundamental pain that we have been hiding behind our food and
weight problem. In order to stop overeating permanently, and
not merely exchange it for another addiction, we need to heal

all our past hurts.

Some of the people I see in my workshops balk when it becomes clear where we are heading. 'But Cherie,' they cry out, 'I didn't ask for the Spanish Inquisition, I didn't come here to have my head shrunk, I just want to lose my problems with food!' What I have been trying to show in the preceding chapters is that even though I can give you short-term tools to help you deal with your overeating, in the long term I truly believe the only permanent solution is to have the courage to delve into your past and confront the demons which drove you to food in the first place. If you do not, they will come back to haunt you, and sooner or later, the old self-destructive pattern around food will reappear.

I think this is the most important message in this book. We need to go back to the place in our childhood where our separation went awry, examine the hurt that was caused, and start to heal the wound. Our task is to bring our wounded inner child out of hiding, and then become a good loving parent to ourselves. We need to confront the pain of the past, and go through a process of grieving over that pain, before we can leave it behind. Only then can we truly free ourselves from the compulsiveness that led to our weight problem.

Grieving is the Healing Feeling

When somebody we love dies we will go through tremendous swings of emotion, including deep hurt, anger, guilt, panic, despair, and depression. This collection of feelings is called grief, and while we are undergoing them we are in the grief process. It is not only death that causes us to grieve, though. The loss of a job, the end of a relationship, a divorce or an abortion, a friend moving far away, or chronic bad health – all of these can make us need to grieve about what has happened to us. We need to kick and scream and talk about what we have lost, over and over again.

The only way out of grief is through it. We can try and skate around, and over and under it, but the only real way out is through. Through the pain, through the anger, through the feeling that our guts have been twisted and our teeth have been knocked out. Not under, not over, but through.

If we do not complete our grieving process, then the blocked feelings accumulate and fester and we live with chronic dis-ease. We may develop an illness, endure constant sadness, and of course we may be driven constantly to overeat. Grieving means expressing the feelings caused by our loss, and sharing our loss with others. Only grieving can help us heal all the symptoms of those blocked feelings.

I have met people who have carried grief inside them for twenty or thirty years, and when they speak about what caused them their pain it is as if it was yesterday. The pain stays as raw and as cutting as the day it was buried. Time does not heal unresolved grief; all time does is that we get used to living flattened and depressed.

If we try and bury our grief and pretend it is not there it will stay inside us, and it will fester and grow and get bigger. It will not go away until we acknowledge it is there and allow it the time and space to leave. Depending on the severity of our loss, the grief work may last a week, a month or a few years, but then *it will be over*. We need to give grief the time it takes to go through it. One day the memory of what happened will just be a memory, and not a twisting knife that we keep buried in our hearts.

People around us may not react well to our grieving if our pain reminds them of their pain, if we speak of somebody who has died, and they remember somebody they have lost. People may want us to pull ourselves together, to be strong, because they are keeping their own lives patched up, and if we cry they feel as if they are falling apart.

After Stephen died I was lucky enough to find Jenny Kander, a skilful bereavement counsellor. In our first few sessions she kept on asking me to tell her about Stephen, what he was like, how he lived, and how he died. It was very painful for me to tell her about him, because I was holding myself taut around the memory of him. It was like walking around trying to balance an egg on the top of my head. I was so afraid to let go, because not only would the egg fall, but the whole of me would crack open and spill out.

As well as speaking about him, Jenny encouraged me to get out old photographs of Stephen and to make a memory album for me and Alan. Speaking about him and making the album enabled me to grieve. My feelings did indeed cause the egg to shatter, but not in the way I had imagined. It is painful to lose somebody you love, and the depth of the pain you feel is the depth of the love. When I released the pain, I also released the love. The first time I really surrendered to the pain, although it was scary and excruciating, it was a tremendous relief. There was also anger. I felt so guilty when I first got angry at Stephen for dying, but Jenny also helped me give licence to my anger. 'How dare he die and leave me alone in Glasgow, how could he leave Alan without a father?' Jenny helped me see that the intensity of my anger was in proportion to my love for Stephen and my need to protect myself. I feel peaceful about Stephen now – I will always love him and I often miss him. I am able to talk about him, think about him, go to our favourite places freely without any restriction, but only because I grieved.

Delving into the Past

Of course it is easy to be aware of the painful events in our adult life which we need to mourn. But we also need to grieve about the hidden pain of our childhood. Buried deep inside us is our 'original pain', the pain which occurred when we lost our real selves, the hurt and anger and despair we lived with when we felt abandoned or neglected or rejected, if our father beat

us, or if our mother lashed us with her tongue. As you begin
to have a relationship with your wounded inner child, as you
begin to recognize how she overeats, so too do you need to let
her tell her story, let her sob out her tears and shout out her
anger.

Your original pain may have been buried for years. With the
buried feelings we have often buried the memories, especially
of our early years. There are techniques for uncovering those
lost memories, for bringing up that lost pain. Later on in this
chapter there are some suggestions about how you can try to
contact your inner child on your own. But you may well find
after a while that you can only get so far by yourself, that
you need outside help. This is why in the Appendix I also
summarize the different therapy options you can explore.

If you have been treated for depression in the past, if
you have had any psychiatric illness, if you are addicted to
alcohol or drugs, or if you suffer from anorexia or bulimia, you
should certainly NOT EVEN ATTEMPT TO DO THIS WORK
WITHOUT BEING SUPPORTED BY A PROFESSIONAL. Nor
should you do so if you were physically or sexually abused as a
child. If at any stage you feel overwhelmed by feelings, that is
the time to seek help too. I could not have done my grief work
on my own and I urge you to seek help if you need it.

Grief from losses in our adult life can sometimes help us to
get in touch with our original pain, as Valerie found when she
could not recover from her divorce. Even though it was four
years after her separation from her husband, and even though
she knew that in many ways her life was a lot more comfortable
– she was dating a nice man, she had moved into a comfortable
flat, she loved having time to see her friends, and to do all the
things she had wanted while she was married – nevertheless she
just could not get over the hurt and anger against her ex-
husband, it ate into her. She would go over and over it in her
mind – his affairs, their arguments, all the times she had sat
waiting for him to come home. Round and round, over and over.
It was only in therapy that she realized that her feelings about

her husband were fuelled by the anger and hurt she had suffered as a child. Her parents used to argue a lot, they were both often out, and they believed in the old saying, 'Children should be seen and not heard.' When she began to grieve for her lost childhood, she was finally able to grieve for her lost marriage, and let go of it.

Things That Go Bump in the Night

It was Janice's day for therapy; we had only half a session left and I was aware that she was heavy with pain. Heavy. I tried gently to make her notice her pain so that she could express it, but whenever she even spoke about it she changed the subject, moved away. She kept on talking about how sad it was that thieves had stolen a painting called *The Scream* by Edvard Munch. There had been a photograph of the stolen painting in the newspaper and Janice could not get this photo out of her mind. I did a visualization exercise with Janice to find out why the theft was bothering her so much, and eventually we found the reason. Janice had grown up in a working-class family with her mother, who was very cold and authoritarian, and her father, who went to work each day and came home at six and read his newspaper, ate his supper and then went to the pub. When Janice was eight she was knocked down by a car and suffered multiple pelvic and leg fractures. She was in bed for six months and then in a wheelchair for a year. The pain was unbearable; she could still remember it as a roaring torture. She remembered that when she cried and sobbed her mother told her to shut up. You are to be silent. Janice quickly learned. To be silent. In the year of excruciating physical pain, she bit into her lower lip and was silent. No cries, no sound. Blood on her lip where she bit so hard to keep out the sound. Janice had always remembered her accident, but she had not remembered how she was forbidden to cry until that day. 'She stole my scream, Cherie,' she sobbed, 'she stole my scream.'

Grief is a process, and it happens in phases and layers. If we imagine grief as an onion, then each layer of the onion needs to be peeled away. We cry the tears caused by the strength of each layer as we go. As we strip away the layers from the outside in, we work backwards in time, towards the core where the most severe hurt and anger is hidden. This is usually the abandonment and abuse we may have suffered as children.

Eating when you are so full you could burst, throwing up when you do eat, and punishing yourself with food, are all the behaviour of your wounded child. It is through this dark pain that you need to move, to find light and happiness again. Grief in all its forms blocks your feelings, so the added bonus of releasing your pain is that you also release your joy, your creativity, your compassion, your ability to love. You will release yourself to be free.

Finding Out Your History

As I mentioned earlier, events from your childhood may be difficult to recollect. Start by piecing your past together – every little thing you can remember is significant. Speak to your siblings, your parents, your schoolfriends, and share memories with them about your childhood. Write down what you remember about your first school, your nursery school. Remember what teachers made an impression on you. Who was your first love? What friends do you remember? Who hurt you? What bad things happened? Find an old family photo album and look through it. Find books that you used to read when you were a child and reread them now. When did your real self become so wounded that she stopped coming out to play?

It is equally important to construct your history around food and eating. If you began eating compulsively when you were a child, you will definitely have been using food as a way to cope with feelings. It will help you to find out why you needed to do that. In the preface of this book I shared with you how I went on my first diet, and what eating patterns I learned from my family. See if you can write a history of your learned eating patterns, dieting history and weight gain. If you like you can use the following questions to guide you:

- Was either of your parents overweight?
- What was your mother's attitude towards her weight and eating? Your father's?
- Were physical appearances very important in your family, and was other people's weight ever a subject of conversation?
- Did your mother or father ever encourage you to think about your weight or comment on the way you looked?
- Did anybody in your family ever ridicule you, or other people, for being fat?
- If you were overweight as a child, how did you feel about the way your family reacted to your weight problem? Did their reaction make things easier or more difficult for you?
- Did your parents eat in a particular way – did they have any peculiar habits around food, or did they like or dislike particular foods?
- Have you inherited any of their food or eating habits?
- What happened when you were hungry when you were a child – did you have to wait for food or was it always available?
- Did you have to finish all the food on your plate, or were you allowed to leave food behind?
- Was food ever used as reward or punishment in your family?
- Were you given food to cheer you up or comfort you?
- Did you ever have delicious treats as a family purely for fun?
- Were you given attention at home or at school for either overeating or undereating?
- Did you ever eat secretly, and why did you? Did your mother or father ever hide foods away? Were sweets and chocolates etc. freely allowed or were they restricted?
- Did food play a central part in your family life – for

example, were there ever any arguments about food, or
was family dinner-time tense and unhappy for any other
reason?

Now turn your attention to the circumstances that led to your
first diet, and the circumstances that surrounded significant
weight gain or loss in your past.

- Think back to the year before you went on your first
  diet. How old were you? Were you really overweight?
- What events had happened leading up to you gaining weight?
  Did you gain weight by reacting to a particular event or had
  you gradually begun to overeat over the years?
- Had something very traumatic or stressful happened just
  before you began to put on weight? (For example, the birth
  of your first child.)

As you write your history, take time out to express the *feelings*
as well as the facts of what you have uncovered. Recalling the
circumstances will bring the memory of the feelings with them,
if you are prepared to face up to them.

Working with Your Inner Child

Imagine a young child aged five or six. You have sole charge
of this child, she is totally at your mercy. She says to you, 'I'm
tired,' and you ignore her. She says to you, 'I need some love,'
and you ignore her; she says to you, 'I want to have some fun,'
and you ignore her. She feels lonely and neglected and sore, and
you ignore her.

It is only when she eats that you suddenly notice she is
there. With venom you turn on her and tell her she has
no willpower, that she is revolting and fat. She feels awful,
and the only place she knows that can help her is the food
cupboard, so she eats some more. You not only scream at
her again, but you put her on a diet. She feels as if food
is all she has, her only protector, her only nurturer, so the

more you tell her she cannot have any, the more she wants it.

You tell her that when she is thin she will be happy, but she does not make the connection between putting on weight and the amount she eats. All she knows is that food dulls the pain she feels. Food somehow relaxes her when she is tense. She thinks that it is food she wants, but the more she eats the hungrier she gets.

A diet is never going to help this child. What she really needs is someone to take her by the hand, talk to her, and explain to her why she wants to eat when she is not hungry. Someone to hold her, to listen to what she has to say, to set limits, and to show her another place to go, when she is desperately rushing towards the kitchen. She needs a new, good loving parent, she needs you.

One day when I was having a conversation with Little Cherie she asked me, 'Why can't you love me, and be nice to me like you are to other people? I wish you would love me like you love them.' She is right. In the past I would always neglect myself, at the expense of others. I listen to Little Cherie now. I have been, and can be, very compassionate, empathic, loving and caring. It is these qualities which I combine to form a nurturing parent for myself. A parent who is wise and gentle as she leads a young frightened toddler out of the kitchen, away from food and towards good loving support. The child is terrified to leave the food so I have to reassure her, teach her gradually how to go through each step along the way. Slowly. Slowly, and with infinite care – remembering always that there is a precious life at stake.

In order to start a new relationship with somebody we need to get to know them. We need to ask them what they are thinking, what kinds of things they like to do. This is the way to begin communicating with yourself; ask your inner child what do you want to do right now, what would make you feel looked after? She will be delighted to answer, and totally thrilled if you pay some attention to her – at last.

Initially it may feel strange to speak with your inner child, you may feel like a fool. But remember that what you are trying to achieve is contact with your real self. You may find it helps initially, to create a visual image of your inner child in your mind by studying photographs of yourself as a child.

The simplest way to communicate with your inner child is to hold a conversation with her in your head. Visualize your loving self, and your inner child, sitting opposite each other and listen to the conversation between the two of them. Because your inner child has been wounded at various ages, she may sometimes be four years old, and at other times an adolescent. So you begin the conversation by asking your child how old she is today. When you are communicating with your inner child, *whatever you hear* will be a true message from within; even if the words sound crazy or ridiculous, just listen, and do your best to understand.

When you speak to your child be as loving as you can – she is very, very needy. Never criticize or scold your child. In order to heal we need to hold and love and put a balm on the scars from the past. Heaping abuse on ourselves totally defeats the object.

A lot of the people I see try to motivate themselves by screaming abuse at themselves. But if you shout at a child, his reaction is often to rebel. The best way to motivate a child is to be loving while setting limits. 'I love you. You have done the best you could in a world that is often hostile and difficult to deal with. Let's talk about this overeating which you tend to do. Maybe we can work out some different ways to help you. I am here for you, my darling, I want to help you. Let's talk about things that really matter to you.' Your inner child will purr with delight.

When you are dialoguing with your inner child, practise the skill of empathic listening. Even though you are speaking to a child, she has the ability to answer you back with an adult understanding. Both of you need to be heard. If my inner child says to me I feel really tired and I answer that I am terribly busy, and then we both continue with our own theme for the conversation, we are not hearing each other. In order really to hear what the other is saying, you need to listen to them carefully, very carefully, both to the content of what they are saying and also to the feeling behind the words.

To show you what I mean here are two conversations with my inner child:

Little Cherie: I am so sick and tired of working.
Cherie: I'm sorry, but I have two meetings this morning and then I have to finish writing the report so I will have to skip lunch.
Little Cherie: I wish I could go to a movie or have a friend around to talk to.
Cherie: I really haven't got time, I wonder if I should cancel going out tonight and then I will be able to fit in more work.
Little Cherie: I keep dreaming about lying on a hammock in the hot sun somewhere.
Cherie: Yes, I will work tonight and then I can definitely fit in that extra work I was planning to take on.
Little Cherie: Oh, well, what can I eat? At least then I can have some fun while she works all the time.

Compare that to a calmer, more focused dialogue:

Cherie: Hello, Little Cherie, what age are you today?
Little Cherie: Eight. I feel kinda funny and strange.
Cherie: You feel a mixture of funny and strange?
Little Cherie: Yes. It is like being in a boat that keeps on going round in circles and if the boat does go slightly forward then it wants to go backwards as well.
Cherie: It sounds as though the boat is confused.
Little Cherie: Yes, the boat is confused and I am on this confused boat. I want to get off.
Cherie: I hear you say that you would like to get off the boat. Can I help?
Little Cherie: Yes, I need you to stop and spend some time with me. We always seem to be rushing here or there. There is always some meeting or someone to see or a group. I need you

to stop and do nice things. Like cycling with Philip on Saturday, that was so nice. We haven't had fun like that for ages.

Cherie: I agree with you, and I would love to have a lot more days like that. Unfortunately I have made a lot of commitments for the next few months and I cannot change them. I wish I could because I feel really tired. I heard you ask me to stop and spend more time with you, I can certainly do that. How about we have a lot more conversations like this and I will fit in as many fun times as I can.

Little Cherie: OK, but you have to promise. I need you for me, and I am tired, really tired now.

Cherie: You are really tired. Would you like to have a rest? We can talk some more later.

Little Cherie: Yes. I want to have a sleep.

Cherie: OK then. Let's speak again later.

Dialoguing in Writing

Another way of dialoguing with your inner child is to write down the conversation between the two of you, to write a letter to your inner child, or to keep a diary. Try using your normal writing hand, when you are being yourself, then switch the pen into the other hand, the hand you usually do not write with, for your inner child. It may feel strange and uncomfortable writing with your left hand if you are right-handed, or vice versa, but the result may surprise you. You will find your inner child hand is messy and almost unreadable, just like a little child's, and the words will come out childish too.

You don't need to limit this exercise to writing, you can also allow your child to further express herself by drawing. If the words get stuck, use your non-dominant hand and draw what it is you are feeling and wanting to say.

Example: MONDAY.

Hi, Little Cherie, how old are you?

Five.

Are you restless? What is it that you feel like doing right now?
I am feeling strange, want to EXPLODE.

Do you want to say a bit more about that?
Ah ha yes inside I feel I feel, I dunno how but I want to explode.

Would it help if you draw this exploding feeling?
Yes!

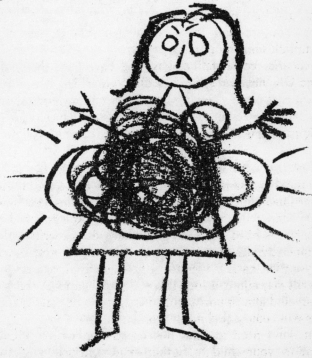

I see you have drawn a picture of a person exploding – does the picture have a title?
The angry person. I AM THE ANGRY PERSON. Angry about Michelle and Suzy.

I AM ANGRRRY!!!

I hear you and I am pleased that you have said why you are so angry. What do you feel you want to do?

I am going to stomp around a bit more because I am so angry.

Go ahead and can we talk some more later.

You can also write letters. This is the first letter I wrote to my inner child. (I felt a bit silly while I was doing it, but now I cannot imagine a life without talking with my inner self every day.)

Dear Little Cherie

After all these years I find you. You have been there all my life and you will be there until I die. You are the most vibrant, mystical part of me. You are my energy and my enthusiasm. It is you who comes out to play, who loves to dance, who runs. You are my centre, you are my emotional being. You are my inner child.

I know that you were neglected and you were ignored and your world is full of fear and pain. I know that you were criticized mercilessly, so much so that you closed yourself into a dark cocoon. You covered yourself over in layers of fat, to keep the world out and to keep yourself in.

I can help you come out into the light. I could not be there for you when you were young, because I was young. In the past I was a parent to you like my parents were to me. So I often abandoned you. I hurt you without knowing I was doing so just as much as they unknowingly hurt me.

You can come over here and be with me, I will not treat you badly any more. You do not need to turn to food, because I will be here for you. I think that you may not trust me, but I will prove to you that you can. It is you that I need to take care of. You are really special, you are fine just the way you are, and I love you very much.

Yours very sincerely
Cherie

This is the reply:

Hello, Hello. I'm pleased you came to find me.

Your inner child may take a while to believe that you are there for her, and that you are willing to be the parent she is desperately searching for. She probably will not trust you immediately.

You will have to work on your relationship, and show her you will take good care of her. Be there for her, and give her the support she needs to grieve and grow. Try to put some time aside each day to dialogue with your inner child. Even if you have the most busy schedule, it helps if you make it a priority.

Affirmations

The way you talk to yourself to a large extent determines how you feel. While you are doing your grieving and healing, remember that you need to start being loving and kind to yourself. In Chapter 7 I talked about doing nurturing things for yourself, and a way to continue that process is to give yourself a daily dose of affirmations.

It is crucial to begin to change that harsh critical voice we are all so familiar with to a more nurturing, esteem-building voice. When you are thinking through your day, look at what you have done and acknowledge yourself for it. If you made a mistake, remind yourself that it is not possible to be perfect, and instead of criticizing yourself, plan how you can prevent the same thing happening again. Stay vigilant to your critical parent voice, and switch it off when it reappears.

When you wake up in the morning, say things that celebrate who you are. Things like:

I like myself just as I am.
I am allowed to make mistakes. Thank goodness I don't

need to be perfect!

I have the courage to change the way that I relate to food. I am learning a new way to eat. I tune into my body's needs. I eat only when I am hungry and stop when I am satisfied.

I choose what I want my life to be. I am becoming more and more aware of my likes and dislikes. I am learning to assert myself. I feel strong. I am in control of my life.

I love and accept myself. I take care of myself. I am aware of my feelings. I am able to experience my pain and be compassionate and kind to myself. I grow stronger every day. I choose to do things that make me happy.

My body has natural strength and ability. I am treating my body with the respect it deserves. I am growing stronger and fitter. I no longer need a covering of fat to hide from the world. My body gives me pleasure. My body deserves to be fed with energy-giving, nourishing food.

I have opinions and I allow others to have theirs. I am a good enough parent and I am a good enough child. I am fine just as I am.

I choose to eat exactly what I want. I remain aware while I am eating. I chew, taste, savour and enjoy everything that I eat. I enjoy nourishing my body. I stop eating when I am satisfied.

I am stepping out. I am sensual and sexual. I am able to let go and enjoy feelings and sensations. I no longer need the protection of an overweight body. I recognize my needs.

I have the knowledge to become naturally slim. My mind is open and receptive to change. I learn and grow all the time. I take risks. I take responsibility for what happens to me.

I am becoming stronger and I am becoming purer. I grow more and more aware of the power I have within me. I do things to the best of my ability. There is nothing to be afraid of. I am special. I am love. I am alive. I am power. I am me. I unconditionally love and accept myself.

Learning from Your Binges

'What may happen to my eating while I am re-parenting my inner child and grieving? When will I lose weight?' you may ask. While you are grieving you may still turn to food to help you over the rough phases. This is the separation phase; you need to let go of food and begin to express your feelings. Keep on giving yourself full permission to eat what you want when you are hungry, and each time you overeat or eat when you are not hungry, ask yourself gently why?

Think back now on the last time you binged or overate. What was going on in the hour before you turned to food? What had happened that day? Were there people around? What were they saying? Or were you alone? Why was it so necessary to eat? Go back to the minute just before you did eat and imagine that instead of eating you did something nurturing and constructive for yourself that did not involve food. What can you learn from this?

Another exercise you can try, to cope with the urge to binge, is to speak directly to the part of your wounded child who overeats.* Close your eyes and imagine that inside of you is a tiny, impish child.

This child loves to eat, and the more she/he grows the more she/he eats. She loves to eat, she lives to eat, she eats and eats and eats and grows bigger and bigger. Picture her growing bigger and bigger. What is the final picture you see? Try drawing the person with your non-dominant hand.

This little monster is the part of your child that has become addicted to food. For her or him food means everything. The need to eat has become like a primal energy, a driving force that flattens every other want or need. Even when you say no, that part of you will always be there urging you, coaxing you,

---

*I got this idea from a wonderful book called *Lighten Up Your Body, Lighten Up Your Life* by Lucia Capacchione.

using a hundred excuses why you should eat even though you are not hungry.

Start a conversation with your addicted child. Begin by asking questions like: 'Who are you?' 'How do you feel?' 'What do you need?' The conversation might flow like this:

I want to eat.

Why do you want to eat? I know you are not hungry.

I want to go and make lots of toast and eat cereal and chocolate. I WANT TO EAT NOW.

I really do not want you to eat when you are not hungry. Can I help? Do you need anything?

Who cares about that, who cares about hungry, ALL I WANT IS FOOD, LOTS OF IT AND I WANT IT NOW.

If I continue to let you eat when you are not hungry we are going to get fatter and fatter.

I don't care about that. Can't you just go and throw up or something? All I want is to eat and eat and eat.

Why do you need to eat so badly?

Why do I need to eat? Well, it is about bloody time that you asked me that. I NEED, DO YOU HEAR ME, I am a NEEDY person.

You need? You are needy.

Yes, I am needy for food, scrumptious, lots and lots of it.

I hear you say that you are needy for food but if you think about it we are not hungry so I would guess that maybe you are needy for something else.

OH, SHUT UP, SHUT UP, I AM GOING TO EAT NOW.

I am not going to let you do that; please tell me what you are really needy for.

I hurt, I really hurt. I just want some peace, there are demons and dragons chewing up my insides and I don't want to be with that. What am I going to do without food? How can I cope without food? Help, help, what do you mean I can't have food? What will I do, where will I turn, I am so lonely, I am so desperate, I need, I need. I am so scared, please let me eat, food makes the fear go away, food dulls the pain. Food calms me down, what will I do without it? Oh no! Oh no, what will I do without food?

I hear you, I feel the pain; you see, you became addicted to food many years ago and I just let you eat whenever you wanted to. You think that food heals the pain, only it doesn't really, it only numbs you for a little while and then you feel worse afterwards.

What do I do then, what do I do?

I can help you. I can hold you when you cry. I can take you places, find you good friends. I know it is scary but there are two of us, and there are other people we can talk to.

Well I'll HAVE TO SEE, I am not quite sure about all this.

I hear your doubts, let's talk again later though, or any time you want to. Let's always talk it through.

Sometimes you will be effective in talking your addicted child out of bingeing, and other times your old way of functioning will take over. Remember, be kind to yourself after a binge, and forgive yourself. Work out how you can handle the situation differently the next time.

You can expect your weight to fluctuate while you still overeat a lot of the time. When you reach a point when you constantly eat only when you are hungry, and stop when you are satisfied, and nourish yourself in other ways when you are not hungry, eventually you will begin to lose weight. I promise.

Reaching Out to Others: You Need a Friend

It is not unusual for people who for years have hidden their feelings behind food, and who have drugged themselves into a stupor through continuous overeating and/or starvation, to find that they have effectively withdrawn from the people closest to them. As we abandon food as our main companion, we need to have and to find a substitute, and we must learn to reach out to others, talk to them, tell them how we feel, ask for their support. I have learned that compulsive eaters are also compulsive givers and rescuers of others, but they find it very difficult to ask for help themselves.

It will be easier if you have a loving partner or family to support you. But you also need friends. In the past, when you looked for friendship and love, you may have done so with your wounded inner child, and found rejection and pain instead. For real, unconditional, loving support, you need to choose your friends with care, and try to find people who understand. You need a place that feels warm, safe and welcoming. The people you choose must really be able to listen to what you are saying. If I say to someone, 'I am so frustrated, at dinner last night I just couldn't stop eating. I knew I was full up, but I just couldn't stop,' I need someone who will understand and empathize, who will say 'It sounds like you had a really difficult time last night, poor you' – not someone who says, 'That's disgusting, why don't you just use your willpower and go on a diet?' The person who is most likely to understand what you are going through and offer you the support and empathy that you need is someone who has suffered herself, perhaps a fellow compulsive dieter or overeater, who like you has decided to learn to deal with her problem, or someone who has already overcome it.

Forming a Support Group

If you do manage to find the right friend, or even a group of friends who are going through the same healing process as you are, you may wish to suggest you form an informal support group, and meet regularly to talk and listen and help each other.

The first support group I started had only three of us in it. I rang up two friends who I knew were also battling with their overeating and we agreed to meet once a week to share our journeys. We decided that each person would have fifteen minutes to speak about what was happening in their lives and then we would all read and do exercises from books which we had found useful.

If you form your own support group it is very important that you take turns to *listen* to each other without interruption. The person who is speaking needs time and space to say what she is going through, she needs to express her feelings. If after someone has shared with the group where they are, the whole group joins in and starts to give them advice about what they should or should not do, it can make the person feel torn and confused, and it just does not work. The best format for a support group is to listen in silence, and then to express and reflect back to the speaker what you see and hear: I notice that your hands are shaking, I feel so sad as you talk about your marriage! You want to allow the person to feel supported while they express their feelings and make their own decisions.

For example, a few nights ago Pam brought this story to the group: 'My mother is dying in hospital, and the staff want me to take her home. I feel dreadful because I do not know if I can cope with that. We cannot afford a nurse and I have three young children so I am run off my feet already. I just don't know what to do.' The group's response was wonderful. Jenny simply told Pam that she had gone through a similar experience recently before her father had died, how she had suffered confusion and guilt about whether to put her father into a nursing home. Tom said that he felt really sad as Pam spoke, and that he noticed she was holding back her tears. As Tom spoke Pam was able to cry, and the people on either side of her put their arms around her. Nobody offered Pam advice as to what she should do. Only Pam can make that decision. But she had shared her feelings with us, which was a relief, and she felt much more supported.

If you form a support group, be really clear about what your intention as a group is. How many weeks you intend to meet for, what you hope to achieve, and what you will do if you need extra help. Keep on assessing if the group is working for you. Do you feel supported? Are you able to express your real feelings? Are you able to be totally honest with each other?

Co-listening

Co-listening is a technique you and your friend may find useful for learning how *really* to listen to each other. I learnt how to co-listen at the Skyros centre in Greece. We were asked to choose a partner, and each pair then withdrew to a quiet place and sat closely facing each other. Then we began to practise really *listening* to each other.

The person who spoke first had ten minutes to talk about what was happening in his life right at that moment. About his feelings, and any decisions he was confused about, about anything that came up in his thoughts, really. During the time your partner was talking, you were not allowed to say one word. If it was my turn to listen I always imagined that I had buttoned my lips closed. It was permissible to nod and say 'uh-huh' or show compassion with your eyes and body language. But absolutely no words. This way you allowed your partner to speak without interrupting his flow of thoughts, and gave him the opportunity to hear what he was thinking himself.

While you were listening you were really concentrating on what the other person was saying. You were looking for themes and feelings so that when he had finished speaking you could give him a brief summary of what he had said, to show that he had been *really* heard, and to reflect back to him the thoughts and feelings he had expressed. No judgement, no advice, just exactly what you had heard in his words. Then it would be your turn to talk, and your partner's to listen, and the process would be repeated.

Unfinished Business

One day you meet a person, you discover that you get along very well, and that you are very similar. You begin to spend time together and a relationship forms. You are really excited, and feel that you have found something special. One day she does something that you don't agree with or like, but you don't say anything. Then you ask her to support you in a time of crisis and she is too busy. A few months down the line you wonder what has happened. The relationship you were so excited about has deteriorated into a tangle.

Imagine that a relationship between two people is like a river which runs between them. When we first meet someone the river is very pure and flows gently and easily. Imagine then that each time something happens between you, if he fails to show up for an appointment, or you betray a confidence or he hates the way you squeeze the toothpaste tube, it is as if you are putting a log in the river. Over the years our pile of logs grows until we have a huge log jam, and our once clear and sparkling river has turned into a stagnant polluted dam! If we want to, we can usually get the river flowing again; we have to figure out which of the biggest logs are causing the obstruction, and work out how to move them.

If you are in a relationship with somebody and you have big logs of unfinished business, that relationship will be contaminated. Unfinished business will make you unhappy, and when you are unhappy you may overeat; and it is much easier to stop overeating if you have love and support from the people around you than it is if your relationships make you hurt and angry. Unfinished business with friends or relations in your past can be part of the wound that you carry inside: naming it and confronting it will help your healing.

Usually the best way to clear the relationship is talk it through. Sit down and tell the other person what is bothering or upsetting you. No matter how well you know somebody you cannot read their thoughts and they cannot read yours. You have to tell them what you are feeling and ask them to explain their feelings. Tell them you have something important to discuss, and arrange an uncluttered time that suits you both. Ask the person to hear you out, to the end of what you have to say, before they have their say. This prevents the conversation from deteriorating into a javelin-throwing match. Keep your adult in the conversation the whole time.

If you have unfinished business to discuss with someone who has died, or whom you no longer see, or if you can't bring yourself to confront the person directly, you can write them a letter (which you probably won't ever send) to get the unfinished burden off your chest. Or take a chair, place it opposite you, and imagine that the person you have unfinished business with is sitting in it. Imagine their face, what they are wearing, and how you feel towards them. And then tell them what you wish to say – it will make you feel better, even though they are not really there.

Overeaters Anonymous

Overeaters Anonymous is a self-help organization based on the same principles as Alcoholics Anonymous and its twelve-step programme. OA groups meet in cities and towns all over the country; they are funded by voluntary donations, and they welcome newcomers. You can find them in the phone book or by asking at your local library. Although I have tried them I have not found OA meetings right for me personally, but a few people whose judgement I really trust have found them enormously helpful. We are all different, so we will find different things helpful.

Therapy

So far all my suggestions for finding support have been of the self-help variety. Nevertheless, many people with an eating problem find that they eventually feel the need to seek out a professional listener. I myself have found my own experience of going to a therapist enormously beneficial, and I would recommend it wholeheartedly. I wish that there wasn't so much stigma attached to therapy in Britain: for some reason, some people here find it a vaguely shameful and embarrassing idea and associate it with 'being a bit mental'. This contrasts sharply with the United States, where having a therapist is as commonplace and unremarkable as having a dentist.

Finding a good therapist can be a bit like shopping for clothes – you need to try on a few before you find one that fits. I found mine on my fourth attempt. The first person I saw was a psychologist. When I told her what I had been going through, cool, well-rehearsed words spilled out of her lipstick. 'You are responding appropriately to what you have gone through,' she said. That was not very helpful, seeing as 'responding' was feeling as if I would like to drive my car over a cliff. The next therapist I found always smelled of garlic, and she would begin to tremble when I cried. Then I saw a man who was sweet and kind, but I always left the therapy session with a feeling that all we had discussed was the weather. So it went on until I found the wonderful Jenny Kander, the bereavement counsellor I have mentioned. In the first session Jenny told me that one day I would find some value out of the things that have happened to me. With her help I managed to say goodbye to Stephen, and come to terms with the shock of his sudden death. I also realized that pain cannot swallow me, that if I give the wound proper attention, it will eventually heal.

When I moved from the city where Jenny was living, I knew I still needed help to work through my original pain, so I wrote down what I was looking for in a therapist:

1. A person who can provide a comfortable, safe environment in which I can express my feelings. Someone who can provide a good sounding board for me, and my ideas. Who will confront my old patterns, but will always provide an overall feeling of acceptance, for who I am, and what I am going through.
2. A person who is wise, and because she or he has travelled further than I have, they can show me the easiest way to go.
3. My wounded inner child feels safe and comforted by that person. That person will always treat my wounded inner child with love and understanding.
4. A person with proper qualifications, and lots of experience.

This time I struck lucky, and found Barbara at my first attempt. With her help, and some group work, I have managed really to see how I was abandoned as a child, and how I now abandon myself. I have learned so much more about myself. It makes for a much easier life for Philip now that he can go to work without me turning into a clinging three-year-old.

Group Therapy

One-to-one talk therapy is very effective, but often, because our memories and the feelings are so far away from us, we may need to use other techniques, to help us further along the road to self-discovery. I think that the most powerful healing work can be done in a group therapy setting. Groups are good because you have the support not only of the therapist, but also of the other members of the group, and listening to their experiences can help to trigger your own feelings. Techniques like psychodrama, gestalt, and art therapy can be very useful too, practised in a group therapy setting with a well-qualified facilitator.

When my son Alan was born he was very premature and weighed only two pounds. He was in hospital for fourteen weeks, during which time he had blood taken twice a day, several lumbar punctures and three operations. The staff in the hospital were friendly, competent and totally unavailable for the emotions that were experienced by the parents of their tiny patients.

The consultant examined Alan one day and then called me over: 'You're a doctor, so I can give you this straight from the shoulder. Your son is spastic.' Reeling from the shock, I walked over to see Alan, who was being attended to by the nurse. She said she was tired and behind in her work, because Alan had needed an exchange transfusion during the night and he had kicked and screamed so much every time the needle went in that it took a whole hour and a half to do it. I looked at her and was horrified to realize that she was actually *complaining* to me. I can still feel my outrage as I write this – was I supposed to feel guilty, was I supposed to comfort her because my son kicked and screamed when she stuck needles into him?

I felt totally numb. In fact I spent the fourteen weeks keeping myself numb. I went to the hospital three times a day every day and cried maybe only a few times. I used my doctor self to remain calm, but inside I was helpless and hurting.

Four years later, I was lucky enough to attend a psychodrama group run by Dr Ari Badaines. On the second day, when one of the participants was speaking about how much she had enjoyed the Winnie the Pooh stories when she was young, I suddenly remembered the poster of Winnie next to Alan's crib in the hospital and before I could think about it I poured out my story. I cried about every needle they stuck into him, I cried about how small he felt when I held him the first time. I cried for the loss of his health, I got angry at the doctor and at the nurse. For an hour the pain and helplessness ripped through me, and I sobbed and screamed. A few hours later I felt as if I had shed a stone in weight. The freedom of letting out the suppressed feeling was like being let out of prison. The pain of watching my child suffering had been weighing me down — expressing it in the group freed me up.

Up until that time, every time I saw a young child running or talking or playing I felt weighed down and heavy with pain. I still cry about Alan, but the pain is what I am feeling in the present moment, not pain cluttered and terrifying by having been held in for years.

Often when I suggest group therapy to people, they tell me they worry they will look silly if they 'break down', and there is no way they can do that in front of other people. I wish I could convince them otherwise. There is no need to feel self-conscious in a group because everyone there has his own reason for being there, and everyone's attitude is therefore non-judgemental. You see, if I am grieving, and I express the feelings caused by my grief, I am *more in control* than if I am running away, hiding from, or overeating because of my pain. When I cry, or get angry, and I do so with awareness, my adult self is giving my inner child permission to be herself. In a way it was easier to pretend I was fine and not hurting about what happened to Alan; I was taking much more of a risk by saying 'I am hurting' than I was by saying 'I am fine'. But finally releasing my pain, I also released my strength, my compassion, and my ability to be vulnerable again.

There is a list of useful contact numbers at the end of this book. The best way to find a professional therapist is by referral. Remember, you may need to interview three or four therapists before you find the correct one. Do not be afraid to leave and find somebody else if it is not working.

Overcoming compulsive eating is a journey, as I have said, and we are all different and so we will all find different things helpful. If something is working for you stick with it, and if it is not, try something else. Only you can decide if you are getting the right kind of help. Keep on checking with yourself: 'Is this working for me? Am I getting enough of the right support? If not, what is missing? Where can I find the right support?' You are entitled to be fussy. It may feel sometimes like you are going three steps forwards and then two steps back, but just keep on going. You will learn, and grow stronger in the process.

I was moved by what Tania said recently at a Weigh Ahead maintenance meeting: 'My life had been wrapped around food and dieting for so long that I had forgotten about my life before I became a compulsive eater. One night at Weigh Ahead when Cherie was asking us if we had ever worked out why we turned to food for comfort, I felt a feeling like icy knives in my gut. I remembered this helpless little girl, crawling to the fridge for ice-cream, as a solution to the constant beatings I got from my mother, and I was absolutely devastated. You will never know the pain I went through. Before I could stop myself I told the group what had happened to me. I was aware they were listening but I was so far away. I told them about the day I hid in the wardrobe and I lay shivering with fear until my mother found me, dragged me out and held my hair as she slapped me several times from side to side. I told them that my father was just as bad as my mother because he *knew* what she was doing yet did nothing.

'It took me a long time to tell my story because the pain engulfed me as I did. My words got choked on and I cried and cried. Cherie suggested that I see a therapist, and two days later I was there telling him the same story. The third time I told anybody about my childhood it was still difficult, but it became easier and easier each time I did. I had this need to share my hurt, and each time I said it, each time I said that my mother beat me, and my father knew and allowed it, it not only became easier to say, it also became less of my fault. I somehow always thought it was my fault, that I deserved the treatment I got from my family. But it was not my fault, I was a helpless child and my mother was emotionally sick and my father was very weak, and I suffered horribly because of them.

'Then I got angry at the two of them, how dare they treat a little child that way. I raved and fumed and wrote letters which I never sent, I imagined myself hitting my mother as she had hit me. Then I noticed something; all the rage and all the pain does have an end. It took me a long time, I still cry and I still get angry, but the pain is today pain and I don't have those icy knives in my gut from my past. When I cry I tell little Tania that she has my full permission to cry, I acknowledge that it must have been hard for her and I say it's OK to cry. It's OK to cry. I am re-parenting myself now, I need not treat myself as my parents treated me. Until very recently that is exactly what I was doing. I mostly eat when I am hungry now. I cannot give myself a new childhood but I can certainly let little Tania have fun and love now. She deserves it, I deserve it, we both deserve it.'

12

Surviving the Long Haul

'If you follow your bliss, you put yourself on a kind of track that has been there all the while, waiting for you, and the life that you ought to be living is the one you are living.'

JOSEPH CAMPBELL

At our first Weigh Ahead meeting newcomers often ask me: 'How long will it take?' I find that question impossible to answer. How long will it take to become naturally slim and find peace? It will take a different amount of time for each and every one of us.

Beth came to a Weigh Ahead course in January 1992. After the first evening she told me that she felt as if a weight had been lifted from her shoulders. 'I will never diet again,' she said. 'I will never go hungry again either. This way of eating makes such sense; from this minute on I will only eat when I am hungry.'

Earlier on that evening I had offered the group a warning. I usually say this twice in any workshop: 'A course like this can make you feel high, and excited. That feeling will last for a while, and eating when you are hungry may be easy for a while. But then it is going to get difficult again. There will be times when you need to say no to foods that you want to eat when you are not hungry. I wish it was plain sailing but I know that it is not. It will take you a while to unlearn the habits of a lifetime. Be patient, and be forgiving of yourself if you lapse back into your old behaviour around food.'

Beth did not hear me say this. Her excitement carried her through for a few months. She ate only when she was hungry, in fact she hardly ever felt hungry, and hardly ate at all, and pounds of weight fell off her. Then she changed jobs, and after her first day at her new job she came home and had a massive binge. She wasn't really worried about it – after all, it was only one binge. But the next day she binged again, and two days after that. Within two weeks she was really struggling.

This, in my opinion, is where Beth's journey really began. When she began eating like a naturally slim person it was easy, because it was a novelty, it was like beginning a new diet. But eventually, Beth's past kicked in and she had to recognize that she needed to undo years of conditioning, years of failure.

The moment that Beth began bingeing and struggling with food again, she had a choice. She could go back to her old habits of dieting and bingeing even though she knew that they made her miserable. Or she could start to work on the underlying reasons of why she overate. Which is exactly what she did.

It was obvious to Beth that she had coped with the stresses and strains of starting a new job by bingeing. But she decided to fill in an eating chart for a couple of weeks so that she could see what other feelings and situations always caused her to dive into food. Once she had it all down in black and white on the chart she began to work out a solution for each individual problem.

Beth decided that she needed extra support in order to express her feelings freely, so she joined a therapy group. For the first time in her life she experienced unconditional acceptance. She could really be herself – happy, angry, sobbing, overeating, frustrated or giggly – and all she got from the group was support, understanding and lots of hugs. Beth also noticed a big difference in her anxiety-related overeating when she practised the deep breathing, visualization and relaxation exercises that she learnt at the group.

But Beth says that an even bigger change happened when she identified her worst enemy. It was herself. The first time Beth became aware of her Critical Parent voice she got a real shock. She discovered that she always spoke to herself in a critical way; she bullied herself, called herself stupid and was never happy with anything that she did. She decided to get to know this critical side of herself so that she could fight back by answering back. She called this critical voice Jezebel, and when she got into the bath and Jezebel began attacking her because of her big thighs and ample fleshy layers she would say: 'STOP. I like myself as I am. I have a lovely soft woman's body.' Whenever she felt guilty or depressed or overly anxious she knew that Jezebel had been having a go at her, so she answered her back, shut her up, and told herself that she was a lovely, courageous, intelligent person. Sometimes she found it was difficult, but every time she caught sight of herself in the mirror she said: 'I like you just the way you are.'

Beth also began to take better care of herself. When she was tired she went to bed early, when she was hungry she ate delicious nutritious food, she bought expensive sexy underwear, went to her favourite movies, organized treats like massage and had a lot of good evenings out with her friends. As she quietened Jezebel down she discovered that she also had a warm, loving compassionate side – which was just as well, because by this stage she had begun to re-parent Little Beth. She had never really been aware before that Little Beth was carrying a childhood full of unhappiness around with her. It took Beth a long time to grieve and heal that childhood wound, but she did it. She kept on going.

Beth's life is so different now. In fact there are days when she does not think of food or her body at all. In the morning she spends some quiet time breathing and meditating, then she gets up, showers, dresses and has her favourite breakfast – muesli with fresh fruit chopped into it, orange juice and two cups of tea. When problems crop up at work she looks at what is happening and searches for a solution. When she gets bored or anxious, or sad or angry, she notices that her first response is to head for food, but because she has acquired the skills, she can now manage her feelings without overeating. When she gets angry she works it out at her exercise class, or she clenches her fists and gives a good yell, right from the bottom of her stomach. When she is sad she cries and asks for lots of hugs. She walks with a spring in her step now, she feels nourished, fit and full of energy. She finds it easier to look in the mirror now, and easy to say: 'I love you, you are an exceptionally special person.'

Beth's weight still fluctuates, but in much smaller increments than in her past. When she exercises regularly and eats nutritious food she is at the lowest point of her setpoint range; when she allows herself to get stressed and anxious she exercises less, eats junk food and her weight goes up to a higher level. But whatever weight she is she accepts herself, she knows that her weight and eating are not a reflection of who she is. Rather, it is her feelings, her friendships, and how she lives her life. She knows she does not have to be perfect. She gets sad, she gets happy, sometimes she has loads of energy and sometimes she gets tired ... All in all, I am pleased to say that she is living happily and emotionally ever after ...

Reaching Your Goal

Have you ever wondered what makes successful people successful? There are examples of successful people all around us. For every Richard Branson, Paul McCartney and Jodie Foster there are thousands of ever-hopefuls who dream about making it. What qualities do some people possess which enable them to realize their potential while others just continue to dream? It isn't as simple as a good education, a high IQ or artistic talent. There are plenty of people with all these qualities who are also struggling along, and do not achieve the success that they desire.

Successful people do not achieve success by accident. What they all have in common is a goal or a vision of the future. To overcome your problem with food you need to form a mental picture of exactly what it is you want to achieve, exactly where it is you are going. You need a goal.

I am writing this last chapter in the university library. It is exam time, and the tension in the air is palpable. When the library closes I am going home. I know how I will get there because I have my car, and a route to follow, from the West End to the south side of Glasgow. If I did not have a clear idea of where I was going when I leave here, then I might get into my car and go in the wrong direction. The only way to get *anywhere*, is first of all to know where it is you are going.

Once you have seen your goal you can begin to map out a route which you can follow. Successful people continuously take positive steps to bring them closer to their goal. They constantly take risks and try out new ideas. Successful people see disasters as a challenge. There are always things that will go wrong, but this brings out the best in the winners because instead of throwing in the towel, they become *more* determined, and they learn from their mistakes. They never lose sight of their goal, and if they veer off course, they immediately take corrective steps.

Years ago this is what I wrote down for my own goal: I

need to eat to live. It is not eating that makes me overweight, it is overeating. I need to understand why and when I overeat so that I can stop. The goal I need to work towards is to eat, with enjoyment, only when I am hungry. In order to eat when I am hungry the best thing I can do for myself is allow myself to get hungry before I eat. While I am eating I need to remain aware of my hunger level so that I can stop eating when I am satisfied. If I find it difficult to stop I need to reassure myself that there is plenty of food available and I can eat again when I am hungry. When I feel the urge to overeat, I must ask myself what is wrong. My compulsion to overeat is a warning signal, and alerts me to my feelings, or to my unsolved problems from my past. I need to continue to address these problems, these feelings, and reach out to others for help if necessary.

As I read this, I can vividly remember what a struggle it was for me at the time to eat when I was hungry, a huge struggle. But I didn't give up and eventually, I achieved my goal.

Long after I had given up dieting, I went to a lunch party on a Sunday afternoon. The host had a reputation as a gourmet chef. The table was laden with food, the sauces were oozing with cream and butter. Dessert was chocolate mousse rich with brandy, and even though there were groans and cheerful complaints about being really full, everybody found room for the fresh, runny Brie and ripe Camembert which followed the meal. I carefully paced myself through the starter, soup and salad, but I knew I had already eaten enough before the main course arrived. The familiar battle started – I wanted to stop eating and yet I could not. I began to withdraw from the conversation. I began to eat faster and faster. Then I noticed what I was doing, and I also noticed what my companions were doing: frolicking and rolling through a massive meal. I suddenly felt left out and angry. The consequence of this big meal for them, I thought bitterly to myself, will be a happy memory; they may perhaps skip dinner, or eat a bit less tomorrow. But if I overeat, I will gain weight! I felt handicapped by my years of dieting, I sensed my fat cells were ready, primed and waiting. One bite, one lick or mouthful of food over my limit and the fat cells would grab it, hold on to it, and send it to my already ample stomach, hips and thighs. By the end of the meal I was in another world: the old world of my compulsive eating. I was going to diet tomorrow. I would skip breakfast, skip lunch and have salad for supper. And the more I planned not to eat the next day, the more I ate that day. The people at the party were now at a distance; I had withdrawn myself from them into the world of compulsive eating. Far away.

I had a sleepless night wondering if I would ever just be able to be free around food. The luncheon had left me feeling really helpless. I reminded myself that I was never going to diet ever again, that I still had a long way to go before I was really a naturally slim person, but that it was not OK for me to give up. Then it hit me. I will always be a compulsive eater. But if I had not been one, I would not be who I am today, and I like what I have become. My chaotic relationship with food, and my wild weight fluctuations, have given me a view of the world which I would never have had. My addiction to food gave me a quest for knowledge. I wanted to understand why I was so helpless around food and so I read and travelled and searched for information. I am a much better person because of all that: it helped me discover my true self, my vulnerability, my strength, my warmth and compassion. When I think back over the past ten years I realize I have been on a continuous journey. Food was never the problem, it was a symptom of the chaos that I felt within myself. It took me years to achieve my goal for my eating, but I believe I have achieved it now – most of the time at least.

Overcoming food addiction is a huge task, a long journey. Like me, you will have good days and you will have bad days. When things go wrong, you need to stop, ask what is happening and choose a new way to proceed towards your goal. Your weight and your mood will fluctuate, up as well as down. When you notice that you are overeating you have a choice. You can just collapse and say, 'Woe is me, I am helpless around food and I'll never be anything but helpless,' or you can acknowledge you are struggling and examine what you need to do to propel yourself forward. Your overeating is a signal that something is wrong; perhaps you could find a support group, change your job, learn about anxiety management, see a therapist.

There is no real end to this journey. Certainly, you can end the nightmare of compulsive obsessing about food and your weight, but there is no real end to the more important journey. Because once you have started, you need never stop growing and learning and reaching your full potential. No end, but so many new adventures: like the first time you go for a walk and notice the birds and the flowers instead of worrying about how fat you are. When you are able to cry the instant you feel pain, when you can feel love for others, and for yourself as well. What a journey.

And I almost forgot to say BON VOYAGE.

Appendix: Your Help Directory

Finding a Therapist

Association of Independent Psychotherapists, PO Box 1194, London
N6 5PW (0171-266 3340)
Individual therapy from £12 to £30 per hour. Also available: super-
vised trainee therapy and couples counselling.
British Association for Counselling, 1 Regent Place, Rugby, Warwick-
shire CV21 2PJ (01788-578328)
Main umbrella organization for counselling in Britain with recognized
code of ethics. £15 to £30 per session for private counselling. For free
local information, phone or write with A5-size s.a.e.
British Association of Psychotherapists, 37 Mapesbury Road, London
NW2 4HJ (0181-452 9823)
Fully recognized professional body with accredited members (largely
in London and south-east). Call or write for details of the Association's
clinical service.

Gestalt Centre, 64 Warwick Road, St Albans, Herts AL1 4DL (01727-864806).

Institute of Family Therapy, 43 New Cavendish Street, London W1M 7RG (0171-935 1651)

Free family therapy may be provided by the NHS. Speak to your GP or local social services.

Institute of Transactional Analysis, PO Box 4104, London WC1N 3XX (0171-404 5011)

Contact for referral to a therapist practising or training in Transactional Analysis. TA's goal is to stop you dealing with the world as you did when you were a child, and to stop the Critical Parent so that you can find your Adult. £30 to £50 for a session lasting 50 minutes; a clinical trainee may charge less.

Westminster Pastoral Foundation, 23 Kensington Square, London W8 5HN (0171-937 6956)

Individual, group and family therapy in 48 affiliated centres across England, Scotland and Wales. Sliding scale fees.

Women's Counselling and Therapy Service, Oxford Chambers, Oxford Place, Leeds LS1 3AX (01132-455725)

Sliding scale of fees according to income – local authority funded.

Women's Therapy Centre, 6 Manor Gardens, London N7 6LA (0171-263 6200)

Young Minds, 22a Boston Place, London NW1 6ER (0171-724 7262)

Puts parents and young people with emotional problems in touch with therapists and counsellors.

Other Sources of Help

Anorexic Aid, The Priory Centre, 11 Priory Road, High Wycombe, Bucks HP13 6SL

Childline (0800-1111)

24-hour free national helpline for children and young people in trouble or danger.

Cruse Bereavement Care, Cruse House, 126 Sheen Road, Richmond, Surrey TW9 1UR (0181-940 4818)

One-to-one counselling in nearly 200 branches nationwide for people upset by the death of someone close. Ring for local branch (for more details, send an s.a.e.).

Eating Disorders Association, Sackville Place, 44 Magdalen Street, Norwich, Norfolk NR3 1JU (01603-621414)

For help and understanding around anorexia and bulimia. Difficult to get through by phone, rather send a large s.a.e. for information about local therapists and support groups. Youth help line only, 01603-765050 (18 years and under 4 p.m.–6 p.m. Monday, Tuesday and Wednesday).

Institute of Psychosexual Medicine, 11 Chandos Street, Cavendish Square, London W1M 9DE (0171-580 0631)

One-to-one and couples counselling on any type of sexual problem, physical or mental. Write with s.a.e. for list of accredited specialists in your area.

Marriage Counselling Scotland, 24 Frederick Street, Edinburgh EH2 2JR (0131-0225 5006)

Marriage and relationships counselling in 15 centres across Scotland.

NAAFA (National Association to Advance Fat Acceptance), PO Box 188620, Sacramento, California 95818 (00 1 916-5586880).

Overeaters Anonymous, see your phone directory for a local number.

Parentline, Westbury House, 57 Hart Road, Thundersley, Essex SS7 3PD (01268-757077)

Helpline network for parents with any difficulties. Also 26 branches open at various times of the day and night. Ring for details.

Relate, Herbert Gray College, Little Church Street, Rugby, Warwickshire CV21 3AP (01788-573241)

Couples counselling in 160 branches across England, Wales and Northern Ireland. Find your local centre in phone book.

Samaritans

If you are feeling desperate and need to talk to someone in confidence, the Samaritans are available 24 hours a day. Local number in phone book.

Youth Access, Magazine Business Centre, 11 Newarke Street, Leicester LE11 5SS

Will provide you with details of free counselling services in your area. S.a.e. appreciated.

Book List

Each of the books on this book list has influenced me in some way. If you want to read further, I suggest you begin with the books that I have marked *.

Bandler, R., and Grinder, J., *Frogs into Princes*, London, Eden Grove Editions, 1990.

Bandler, R., *Using Your Brain for a Change*, Utah, Real People Press, 1985.

Berne, E., *Transactional Analysis in Psychotherapy*, London, Souvenir Press, 1975.

Bradshaw, J., *Healing the Shame That Binds You*, Florida, Health Communications, 1991.

*Bradshaw, J., *Homecoming: Reclaiming and Championing Your Inner Child*, London, Piatkus, 1991.

Bradshaw, J., *Creating Love: The Next Great Stage of Growth*, London, Piatkus, 1993.

Bruch, H., *Eating Disorders*, London, Routledge & Kegan Paul, 1974.

Campbell, J., *The Power of the Myth*, London, Doubleday, 1989.

*Capacchione, L., *Lighten Up Your Body, Lighten Up Your Life*, California, Newcastle Publishing Co., 1990.

Capacchione, L., *Recovery of Your Inner Child*, New York and London, Simon & Schuster, 1991.

Chernin, K., *The Hungry Self: Women, Eating, and Identity*, New York, HarperCollins, 1994.

Chernin, K., *Womansize: The Tyranny of Slenderness*, London, Women's Press, 1983.

Dana, M., and Lawrence, M., *Women's Secret Disorder: A New Understanding of Bulimia*, London, Grafton, 1988.

Dickson, A., *The Mirror Within: A New Look at Sexuality*, London, Quartet Books, 1985.

Dickson, A., *A Woman in Your Own Right: Assertiveness and You*, London, Quartet Books, 1982.

Eichenbaum, L., and Orbach, S., *Understanding Women*, London, Penguin Books, 1985.

Erikson, E., *Childhood and Society*, London, Paladin, 1977.

Estes, C. P., *Women Who Run with the Wolves: Contacting the Power of the Wild Woman*, UK, Rider, 1993.

*Forward, Dr S., *Obsessive Love: When It Hurts Too Much to Let Go*, London, Bantam Books, 1993.

*Forward, Dr S., *Toxic Parents: Overcoming Their Hurtful Legacy and Reclaiming Your Life*, London, Bantam Books, 1991.

Freed, A. M., *Transactional Analysis for Teens and Other Important People*, California, Jalmar Press, 1976.

Gawain, S., *Living in the Night: A Guide to Personal and Planetary Transformation*, London, Eden Grove Editions, 1988.

Gilbert, S., *The Psychology of Dieting*, London, Routledge, 1989.

Glouberman, D., *Life Choices and Life Changes Through Image Work: The Art of Developing Personal Vision*, London, Aquarian Press Ltd., 1992.

Hay, L., *You Can Heal Your Life*, London, Eden Grove Editions, 1988.

Hillman, C., *Recovery of Your Self-Esteem: A Guide for Women*, New York and London, Simon & Schuster, 1992.

*Hirschmann, J., and Munter, C., *Overcoming Overeating*, UK, Mandarin, 1990.

*Jeffers, S., *Feel the Fear and Do It Anyway*, London, Arrow Books, 1991.

Jones, M., *Secret Flowers: Mourning and Adaptation to Loss*, London, Women's Press, 1988.

*Kano, S., *Never Diet Again*, London, Thorsons, 1990.

Lerner, H. G., *The Dance of Anger: A Woman's Guide to Changing the Patterns of Intimate Relationships*, London, Pandora Press, 1992.

Levine, S., *Who Dies?: An Investigation of Conscious Living and Conscious Dying*, Bath, Gateway Books, 1988.

Levine, S., *Meetings at the Edge*, Bath, Gateway Books, 1992.

Meadow, R. M., and Weiss, L., *Women's Conflicts About Eating and Sexuality: The Relationship Between Food and Sex*, New York, Harrington Park Press, 1992.

Miller, A., *Banished Knowledge: Facing Childhood Injuries*, London, Virago, 1991.

Miller, A., *For Your Own Good: The Roots of Violence in Child-rearing*, London, Virago, 1987.

Miller, A., *The Drama of Being a Child*, London, Virago, 1987.

O'Garden, I., *Fat Girl: One Woman's Way Out*, New York, Harper-Collins, 1993.

Ogden, J., *Fat Chance!: The Myth of Dieting Explained*, London, Routledge, 1992.

Orbach, S., *Fat is a Feminist Issue*, London, Arrow Books, 1988.

Parks, P., *Rescuing the Inner Child: Therapy for Adults Sexually Abused as Children*, London, Souvenir, 1990.

Proto, L., *Who's Pulling Your Strings?: How to Stop Being Manipulated by Your Own Personalities*, London, Thorsons, 1989.

Robbins, A., *Unlimited Power*, London, Simon & Schuster, 1989.

*Roth, G., *Feeding the Hungry Heart: The Experience of Compulsive Eating*, London, Penguin Books, 1983.

*Roth, G., *Breaking Free from Compulsive Eating*, New York, Signet, 1984.

*Roth, G., *Why Weight?: A Guide to Ending Compulsive Eating*, New York, New American Library, 1989.

*Roth, G., *When Food is Love: Exploring the Relationship between Eating and Intimacy*, London, Piatkus, 1992.

Rowe, D., *Wanting Everything: The Art of Happiness*, London, Fontana, 1992.

*Sandbek, T. J., *The Deadly Diet: Recovering from Anorexia and Bulimia*, California, New Harbinger Publications, 1986.

*Sanders, T., and Bazalgette, P., *You Don't Have to Diet*, London, Bantam Press, 1994.

Schwartz, B., *Diets Still Don't Work*, Texas, Breakthru, 1990.

Siegel, B. S., *Love, Medicine and Miracles*, London, Arrow Books, 1989.

Skynner, R., and Cleese, J., *Families: And How to Survive Them*, London, Mandarin, 1993.

Steinem, G., *Revolution from Within: Book of Self-Esteem*, London, Corgi, 1993.

Stewart, I., and Joines, V., *Transactional Analysis Today*, London, Lifespace, 1987.

Stone, H., and Winkelman, S., *Voice Dialogue: A Tool for Transformation*, California, DeVorss and Co., 1985.

Stone, H., and Winkelman, S., *Embracing Ourselves: The Voice Dialogue Manual*, California, New World Library, 1989.

Stone, H., and Winkelman, S., *Embracing Each Other: Relationship as Teacher, Healer and Guide*, California, New World Library, 1990.

*Whitfield, C. L., *Healing the Child Within: Discovery and Recovery for Adult Children of Dysfunctional Families*, Florida, Health Communications, 1991.

Whitfield, C. L., *A Gift to Myself*, Florida, Health Communications, 1991.

*Williamson, M., *A Return to Love: Reflections on the Principles of a "Course in Miracles"*, London, Aquarian Press Ltd., 1992.

Wolf, N., *The Beauty Myth*, London, Vintage, 1991.

Woodman, M., *The Owl Was a Baker's Daughter: Obesity, Anorexia Nervosa and the Repressed Feminine*, Canada, Inner City Books, 1982.

If you can't find any of these books in your local library or bookshop, try the following:

Karnac Books, 118 Finchley Road, London NW3 5HJ (0171-431 1075) and 58 Gloucester Road, London SW7 4QY (0171-584 3303).

Compendium, 234 Camden High Street, London NW1 8QS (0171-485 8944).

Book Service By Post Ltd., PO Box 29, Douglas, Isle of Man 1M99 1BQ (01624-675137), who will order books published in the UK and the USA.

Index

If you wish to write to Cherie Martin, she will be pleased to receive your letter, but she regrets that she cannot reply personally to each one.

For information about the Weigh Ahead workshops, please send a large stamped addressed envelope to:

Cherie Martin
Weigh Ahead
P.O. Box 5108
Busby
Glasgow G76 8HT